AF880130

Kashmir & International Armed Conflict

Nasir Qadri
Musaib Manzoor

Kashmir & International Armed Conflict

ELIVA PRESS

ISBN: 978-99993-1-239-4

© Eliva Press Global Ltd. part of Eliva Press S.R.L., 2023
© Nasir Qadri, Musaib Manzoor

Cover Design: Eliva Press
Cover Image: www.ingimage.com
Email: info@elivapress.com
Website: www.elivapress.com

This Eliva Press imprint is published by the registered company Eliva Press Global Ltd. part of Eliva Press S.R.L. Publishing Group

The registered company address is: Pope Hennessy Street Level 2, Hennessy Tower Port Louis, Mauritius
Eliva Press S.R.L. Publishing Group legal address is: Bd. Cuza-Voda 1/4 of. 21, Chisinau, Moldova, Europe

No part of this book may be reproduced or utilized in any form or by any means, electronic or mechanical, including photocopying, recording, or by any information storage and retrieval system, without permission in writing from Eliva Press. Any brand and product names mentioned in this book are subject to the trademark, brand, or patent protection and are trademarks of their respective owners. The use of brand names, trade names, product names, product descriptions, is in no way implies that such names may be regarded as unrestricted by trademark and brand protection laws and thus may be used by anyone. The opinions and views expressed are exclusively those of authors/contributors and in no way the editors or publisher is responsible.

All rights reserved.

Kashmir and International Armed Conflict

By Legal Forum for Kashmir

Srinagar, IOK / Islamabad, Pakistan

Forward:

The law of armed conflict is a key element of the global legal order, yet it finds itself in a state of flux created by the changing nature of warfare and the influence of other aspects of international law. The *Discussion Series on Kashmir and International Armed Conflict* provides a unique perspective on the field covering all key features of the law, as well as identifies the development and often contentious areas of interest pertaining to the Kashmir struggle.

Ever since the end of the second World War, the geopolitics and order of the world have undergone significant changes, particularly after the collapse of the Soviet Union over three decades ago, and the rise of China in the past decade. Yet, two tragedies, namely in Palestine and Kashmir, have been enduring and unfolding due to the nature of the protagonists who refuse to abide by international law or recognize their culpability in perpetuating these devastating conflicts. What made the struggle for freedom and self-determination in these two intractable cases even more challenging, was the failure of the so-called international community, particularly great powers, to hold Israel and India accountable for the tragic consequences of their military occupation and political obstinance.

While there are many striking similarities between both conflicts, the Palestinian struggle is much more widely known and written about than the struggle in Kashmir. Thus, this volume serves as an excellent introduction and primer to the Kashmir struggle particularly to those who lack the necessary background needed to understand the historical nature and evolvement of the conflict, and be motivated to actively work for ending the war, the injustice, the suffering, and the violation of human rights perpetuated against the Kashmiri people on a daily basis

This volume is a compilation of outstanding analyses and essays presented by eighteen renowned scholars and experts in a Webinar Series organized by LFK. Each chapter walks the reader through a unique narrative of the Kashmir story using the optic of legal framework and vivid human passion. What makes it stand out is its remarkable approach in not only exposing the unconscionable atrocities and catastrophic consequences carried out by the occupation and militarization of Kashmir, but also by offering a wide range of sensible policy recommendations and practical suggestions to peacefully resolve the decades-old tragedy. The methodology used by the authors is scholarly and figurative, and employs both qualitative and quantitative approaches.

As someone who has been for decades a keen observer of many struggles around the word for justice, freedom, and dignity, I found the essays of this volume extremely valuable and useful for both, the experts and laypeople. They are exceptionally well written as they collectively capture the most important aspects and arguments for the struggle for self-determination in Kashmir. After reading the book, any fair-minded, good-hearted, and humane individuals would have no choice but to lend their strong support to the just cause of the people of Kashmir to live in freedom and dignity in their own country under a genuine democratic system without fear or want. The case for such peaceful and just outcome has been aptly laid out in this volume. And there lies its remarkable strength and lasting impact.

Prof. Sami A. Al-Arian
Center for Islam and Global Affairs,
Istanbul Zaim University, Turkey
January 29, 2021

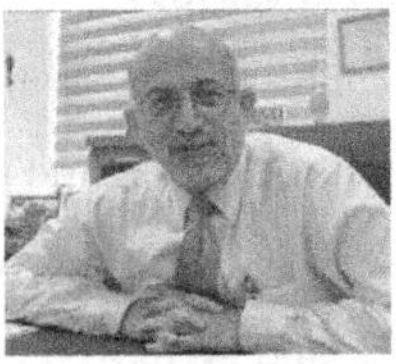

List of contributors:

Dr Muhammad Mushtaq:

Dr Muhammad Mushtaq is Director General of Shariah Academy, Pakistan. He has written his thesis on Use of Force for Right to Self-determination under International Law, Modern and Islamic perspective. Besides, Dr Mushtaq is author of five books and has written dozens of Articles on Laws of War.

Ambassador Ashraf Qazi

Ambassador Ashraf Qazi is former diplomat. He has served in the US and many other regions as Ambassador of Pakistan

Dr Ghulam Nabi Fai

Dr Ghulam Nabi Fai is global Kashmiri diaspora leader and secretary general of US-based World Kashmir Awareness Forum.

Justice Ali Nawaz Chowhan

Justice Chowhan is former Judge at Hague and Chief Justice of Gambia. He is presently Honorary Chairman LFK

Dr. Niaz Shah

Niaz A. Shah is barrister and professor in law. He is author of several book including Islam and the law of armed conflict. He is one of the general editors of journals of international humanitarian legal studies. He also worked as a protection assistant for

UNHCR and remain consultant of UNICEF. He is currently working on research project Application of International Human rights law in Muslims states.

Ambassador Abdul Basit

Abdul Basit, a retired Pakistani diplomat who served as a former High Commissioner of Pakistan to India in New Delhi. He was also appointed as Ambassador to Germany. During his career he was posted at Moscow, New York, sanna and London.

Dr. Patricia Hobbs

Patricia Hobbs is lecturer in law, Brunel University. Her doctoral thesis focused on the relationship between Rome statute and the principle of state sovereignty. She has been regular judge in mooting competitions organized by Brunel University

Prof. Abdul Rauf Khatana

Abdur Rauf Khattana is Assistant Professor of Law, LL.M in Human Rights, Conflict and Justice (SOAS, UK), MA in Philosophy (University of Peshawar).

Farzana Yaqoob

Farzana Yaqoob is the Founding Member of the Asia Institute of Public Policy and is a Policy Advisor for AGAHI. She formerly served as Minister for Social Welfare and Women Development in Azad Jammu and Kashmir, having been elected in 2011. She is also an Eisenhower Fellow (2016); her focus during the fellowship was on conflict resolution and climate change mitigation strategies.

Prof. Sikander Ahmed Shah

[1] Professor Sikander Shah is a pioneering member of the Shaikh Ahmad Hassan School of Law, LUMS. Professor Shah served as the Legal Advisor to the Ministry of Foreign Affairs, while he was on sabbatical in 2012-2013. Professor Shah's teaching and research

interests are focused on Public International Law, International Human Rights Law, International Humanitarian Law, Corporate Governance and Constitutional Design.

Sami-ur-Rehman

Sami ur Rehman is assistant professor at shariah academy.

Raja Sajjad Khan

Raja Sajjad Khan is director Jammu Kashmir Liberation cell, Government of Azad Jammu Kashmir and PHD scholar IIUI.

Catherine Constantinides

Catherine is an international speaker. A Humanitarian, Human Rights Defender and Climate, environmental & Social Justice Activist.

Hassan Aslam Shad

Hassan Aslam shad is Harvard Law School graduate with expertise in international law and corporate law with a heavy focus on the Middle East. Op-ed writer on law fare themes, international law, geo-strategy and international relations. Now working as Legal Director at CMS McKenna, Oman. Mr. Shad also had the distinctive honor of being the first person from Pakistan to intern at the office of the president of the international criminal court The Hague.

Afzal Khushal Khan

Afzal khushal is graduate of the University of Glasgow in international law, his thesis was on Kashmir conflict with an entire international law perspective.

Dr. Junaid S. Ahmed

He is a PhD scholar and professor of politics and islamophobia studies, visiting faculty university of Leeds research fellow center for Islam and global affairs Istanbul and the Director of the center for Muslim world studies and professor of religion and global politics.

Iman Zainab Hazir Mazari

Iman mazari, LLM in international law and legal studies, university of Vienna, an international law researcher and an activist. She is also a Founding partner, MH Advocates & Legal Consultants

Muhammad Shoaib

Muhammad Shoaib is LLM from Bahria University Islamabad under the scholarship of ICRC and his research mainly revolves around role of civilians during armed conflict. Mr. shoaib has wrote articles related to Kashmir, cpec, secp, genocide and war crimes.

Oves Anwar

Mr. Anwar is Director of Research society of International Law (RSIL). He holds an LL.M with distinction from the School of Oriental and African Studies, UK, and an LL.M in International Legal Studies from the University of Vienna, Austria. He has also earned a Diplôme d'université in International Nuclear Law from the International School of Nuclear Law, University of Montpellier, France.

Preface

From 4th September – 23rd November 2020, the Legal Forum for Kashmir (LFK) virtually hosted distinguished international law scholars, diplomats and practitioners to participate in a discussion examining the nature of armed conflict in Indian-occupied Kashmir (IOK). Panelists discussed the disputed status and the ongoing armed conflict in the region. The discussions spread across six panel discussions.

The summaries of the discussions were prepared by Bakht Fatima, Tayyaba Sultana, Maria Awan and Muhammad Shehryar, all of whom are lawyers. The synopses recapitulate the highlights of each speaker presentations.

The LFK is indebted to all the distinguished speakers and panelists for their valuable time and participation.

We also thank scholar-activist Ibn Sina and Islamabad-based Usama for their continuous support during the sessions, as well as editing the discussions book on International Armed Conflict and Kashmir (IAC&K).

This book would not be possible without the valuable back-end support by Umar Bhat, Zain ul Abideen and the LFK's law fare division.

We hope this endeavor will add to, and help shape the debate on evolving legal issues regarding the Kashmir dispute.

Nasir Qadri Advocate

Executive Director LFK

Introduction

Advocate Nasir Qadri

The Law of Armed Conflicts (LOAC) or International Humanitarian Law (IHL) plays an important role in conflicts around the world. The conflict in UN-recognized disputed territory of Indian-occupied Kashmir (IOK) gives us a history riddled with war, destruction, armed conflicts and widespread violations of IHL.

To properly locate and analyze human rights violations in the IOK, the history of the dispute, the level of intensity, and the parties involved must be estimated. A change in the current situation allows the inspection of conflicts of an international nature – International Armed Conflict (IAC).

The IAC, as defined under Common Article 2 of the Geneva Conventions of 1949, refers to hostilities involving "High Contracting Parties", essentially specifying nation states. The IAC includes "all cases of declared war or any other armed conflict which may arise between two or more of the high contracting parties, even if the state of war is not recognized by one of them."

Thus, the threshold of an IAC is low and its existence is determined by the nature of involving parties, not by the subjective intent of the belligerents or duration and intensity of the conflict.

In this context, India and Pakistan being the two high contacting parties to the dispute have been engaged in an international armed conflict over the status of Jammu and Kashmir since their inception.

So far, the two parties have fought three major wars over Kashmir, including the Indo-Pak War of 1947–48 and 1965.

Besides, Kashmiris are struggling for their right to self-determination (RSD) as guaranteed by United Nations for the last seven decades.

The government of India tries to downplay the conflict, despite the fact that thousands of Kashmiris have been killed, tortured, raped, arbitrarily detained, subjected to enforced disappearances and their properties being damaged.

On the other hand, there is no end to ceasefire violations, essentially by India, along the Line of Control (LOC), which is also seen as "*war by other means*"[1] and are increasing since 2013.

Dietrich Schindler, a member of the International Committee of the Red Cross (ICRC) Legal Commission, argues that "*the existence of an armed conflict within the meaning of Article 2 common to the Geneva Conventions can always be assumed when parts of the armed forces of two States clash with each other." He adds that "any kind of use of arms between two states brings the Conventions into effect.*"[2]

Hence, the nature of Kashmir conflict brings both states under the obligations affirmed by the IHL, as both India and Pakistan are parties to the four Geneva Conventions of 1949.

In addition, they are also bound by the Customary IHL.

In this context, the magnitude and perpetuity of the IAC between the two high contracting parties, incurring social, physical and material losses to the people of IOK specified as protected under Geneva Conventions – who do not or cease to be part of hostile activities – call for applicability of the IHL provisions, thereby invoking the commission of war crimes in the Kashmir conflict.

---

[1] Christophe Jaffrelot, "*Ceasefire Violations in Kashmir: A War by Other Means?,*" *Carnegie Endowment for International Peace*, October 24, 2018. https://carnegieendowment.org/2018/10/24/ceasefire-violations-in-kashmir-war-by-other-means-pub-77573

[2] Dietrich Schindler, *The Different Types of Armed Conflicts According to the Geneva Conventions and Protocols*, *Collected Courses of the Hague Academy of International Law*, Vol. 63, No. II (1979): 131.

The graph shows the total fatalities during the armed conflict in Indian-occupied Kashmir from January 2010 - June 2020.

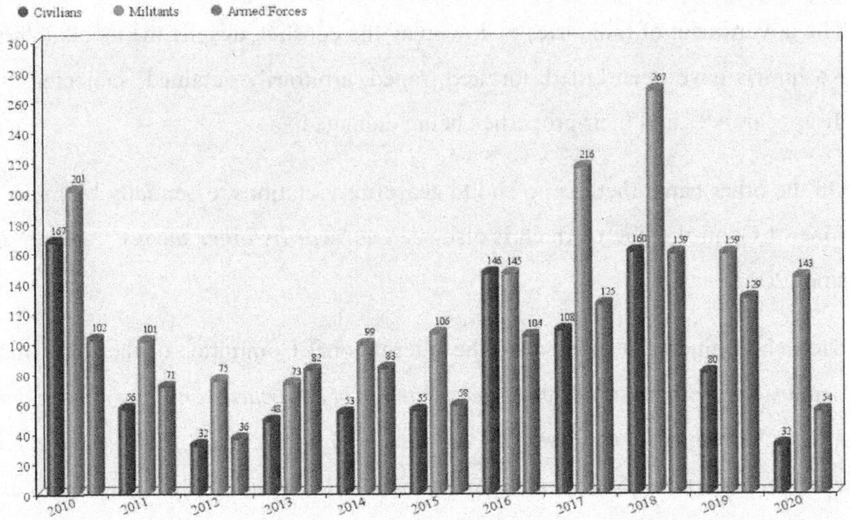

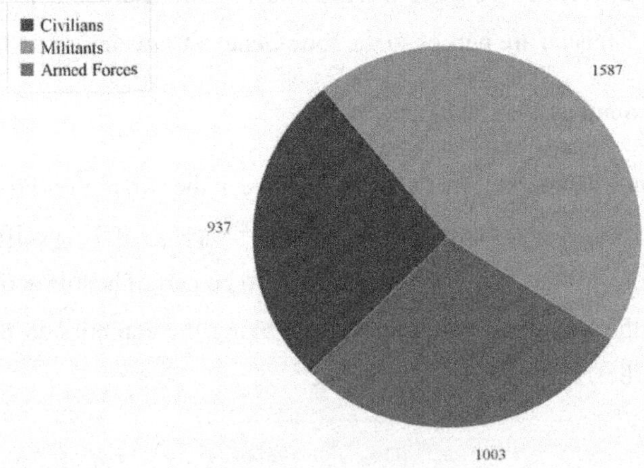

Source: JKCCS

List of Abbreviations

AFSPA	Armed Forces Special Power Act
CAT	Convention Against Torture
DAA	Disturbed Areas Act
EU	European Union
HM	Hizbul Mujahideen
IAC	International Armed Conflict
ICC	International Criminal Court
ICL	International Criminal Law
ICRC	International Committee of the Red Cross
IHL	International Humanitarian Law
IOJK	Indian Occupied Jammu & Kashmir
IOK	Indian Occupied Kashmir
J&K	Jammu and Kashmir
LFK	Legal Forum for Kashmir
LOAC	Law of Armed Conflict
LOC	Line of Control
NIAC	Non- International Armed Conflict
OIC	Organization of Islamic Cooperation
PSA	Public Safety Act
UN	United Nations
UNHRC	United Nations Human Rights Commission
UNGA	United Nations General Assembly
UNSC	United Nations Security Council

Session I

International Armed Conflict and Kashmir's Struggle for Right to Self-Determination

Dr Muhammad Mushtaq Ahmad[3]

I will try to explain the unceasing International Armed Conflict in Kashmir. I shall chiefly focus on International Humanitarian Law as per the Geneva Conventions, Additional Protocols, and some general principles of International Humanitarian Law.

The entire issue revolves around the right to self-determination. One cannot help but wonder: why the international community has not been fulfilling its responsibilities in this regard?

To quote Woodrow Wilson:

"We believe these fundamental things: First that every people has a right to choose the sovereignty under which they shall live; ... Second, that the small states of the world have a right to enjoy the same respect for their sovereignty and for their territorial integrity that great and powerful nations expect and insist upon. And, third, that the world has a right to be free from every disturbance of its peace that has its origin in aggression and disregard of the rights of peoples and nations"

These three points give us the basic idea of self-determination. They also explain that peace is not possible if you continue to deny the right of self-determination to peoples and nations. This is exactly what Woodrow Wilson explicitly stated in his speech when he said, and I quote, *"No peace can last, or ought to last, which does not recognize and*

[3] Dr Muhammad Mushtaq is Director General of Shariah Academy, Pakistan. He has written his thesis on Use of Force for Right to Self-determination under International Law, Modern and Islamic perspective. Besides, Dr Mushtaq is author of five books and has written dozens of Articles on Laws of War.

accept the principle that governments derive all their just powers from the consent of the governed, and that no right anywhere exists to hand peoples about from sovereignty to sovereignty as if they were property."

Thus, people are not commodities that can be handed over from one sovereign party to another. This is the crux of the matter. In his famous 14 points, Woodrow Wilson talks further about the right to self-determination for certain people, of course, in the European context. One may also refer to the ideas of Lenin who talked about self-determination not only for the Europeans, but for Asians, Africans, and even the people of Soviet Union.

Article 72 (of the Soviet Constitution) acknowledged the right of the people to secede – the right of the constituent republics to disassociate from the union – although, practically improbable. But, the very idea that these constituent republics could secede from the union was fascinating; and disturbing as well, for some of the people. And that is why, the US secretary of the state at that time deemed it destructive to the stability of the future world, if right to self-determination was to be enjoyed by the colonial states.

Here lies the problem: When it comes to European powers, and when it comes to people in the western world, there is all support for the right to self-determination. However, when one talks about the right to self-determination for colonial world and for the colonial populace, who are under alien domination, the same western powers brand it disturbing and destructive to the stability of the world. This is indeed sad on the part of so-called champions of democracy.

Nonetheless, I would like to come to the *Atlantic Charter* of 1941, which the then president of the United States and the prime minister of the United Kingdom adopted on August 14, 1941.

Among other things, it says, and I quote, *"They desire to see no territorial changes that do not accord with the freely expressed wishes of the peoples concerned."* Interestingly, later on, Winston Churchill expressed its exclusiveness for Europe only. This is the kind of double standards we are bringing to light.

One can see the same bias during the drafting of the UN Charter. Belgium and some other western powers specifically objected to these provisions. Regardless, the right to self-determination and principle of equal rights were included in Article 1 and Article 2 of the foundational treaty.

Much has been said about the resolutions of the UNSC. I will refer here to the resolutions which were adopted by the UN General Assembly, more importantly, resolution number 1514, adopted in 1960, during the 25th year of the Declaration on Granting Independence to Colonial Territories and Peoples. The whole decade was termed as the decade of decolonization.

Another significant resolution was that of 1970, resolution number 2625, the Declaration on Principles of International Law, Friendly Relations and Cooperation among States. This resolution also mentions the right to self-determination. The United Nations General Assembly (UNGA) adopted another important resolution in 1974, resolution number 3314, the Adoption of Definition of Aggression. This is important because here the General Assembly was trying to come up with a consensus definition of aggression and even here, in their consensus definition of aggression, they excluded the struggle for self-determination.

People sometimes confuse the struggle for self-determination with that of terrorism. Resolution number 3034 of 1972 talks about Measures to Prevent International Terrorism. It delineates terrorism as acts that endanger or take innocent human lives, or jeopardizes fundamental freedom. It further discussed that underlying causes of these forms of terrorism and acts of violence lie in misery, frustration, grievance and despair, which consequently cause some people to sacrifice human lives, not excluding, their own in an attempt to affect radical changes.

Hence, the UNGA recognised that it is utter misery, frustration, grievance, and despair, and denial of fundamental freedom that pushes a man or woman to sacrifice his or her own life in an attempt to bring change.

Another interesting resolution passed by the UNGA in 1984 against state terrorism again reaffirmed the obligation to respect the right to self-determination.

All in all, on the one hand, there were developing countries which were recently decolonized and protesting for the right to self-determination. And on the other, there were western powers, which had colonized them. The western power centres were trying to dilute the right to self-determination by stressing upon stability. This is evident even when the Additional Protocol to the Geneva Conventions was adopted in 1977.

Article 1, sub Article 4 of the Additional Protocol is important for us. It includes *Armed Conflicts* in which people are fighting against colonial domination, alien occupation, and racist regimes. The exercise of the right of self-determination is enshrined in the charter of the UN and the Declaration on Principles of International Law concerning friendly relations and cooperation among states in accordance with the Charter of the United Nations. So, referring to the 1970 resolution, as well as to the UN charter, this Article says that people who fight against colonial domination, alien occupation, and racist regimes for exercising their right to self-determination, for such people, this additional protocol is applicable. This Additional Protocol, Article 1, sub Article 4, thus, acknowledges that the Kashmir issue is an International Armed Conflict. However, it is well known among the academia, as well as the international community that western scholars, at least, a large group of them, has been persistently trying to undermine the significance and the application of this particular article.

Even if you look at the commentary of the ICRC, there are opinions about confining the operation of this article to the colonial context.

During the First World War, and between the two world wars, the talk about self-determination was exclusive to colonial mandate system. It was introduced by the League of Nations. But, when the above stated resolutions, and many other such resolutions, were passed by the UNSC, it was perhaps the first time that a right of self-determination was taken out of the particular colonial context. This generalized and globalized the Palestinian, issue and the issue was taken further after the disintegration of the former Yugoslavia in the 1990s.

Now an important issue in this regard for international humanitarian law perspective is that Article 2, common to the four Geneva conventions, specifically says that if there is occupation, there is International Armed Conflict. The four Geneva Conventions apply to the either situation: complete occupation and partial occupation. It says that even if there is no resistance to this occupation, the occupation itself is enough to constitute an International Armed Conflict.

Dr. Ijaz Hussein, a scholar, has written a well-researched book, *Kashmir Dispute, An International Law perspective*. He explains in detail why the accession was not legal under international laws, why the Maharaja Hari Singh did not have the power to do this, and even if he had the authority, what were the circumstances in which he acceded to the Indian Union, and why they could not be considered to be valid: coercion since Indian troops had already landed there, among other legal arguments. He has encompassed relevant details of the legal principles involved here. Thus, once we establish that there is occupation, either partial or complete, even if there is no resistance, this is an International Armed Conflict, and indeed a case of prolonged occupation.

One of the problems associated with prolonged occupations is that people tend to forget that they are unjust and forceful occupations. Although, legally it is an occupation, it is illegal. Sooner or later, the occupant has to leave. And once you establish that, there are many instruments which become significant. For example, the Fourth Geneva Convention talks about the duties of the occupying power, the obligations and the rights of the people in the occupied territory.

There are several other significant international documents in this regard, as well. For example, the International Court of Justice's advisory opinion on the construction on the legality of occupied Palestinian territory, where it has enumerated all the legal consequences from the perspective of human rights law, humanitarian law, and criminal law as well as from the perspective of occupational law.

Unfortunately, people have considered the dispute as a dispute between Pakistan and India only, and they have overlooked the fact that the state of Jammu and Kashmir is occupied by India, and there is a ceaseless, on-the-ground struggle for self-determination. The issue remains unresolved, to date.

The world needs to be reminded time and again of the origin, and that the issue remains unsettled. The agenda remains incomplete. There is no escape from the fact that Kashmir is an occupied territory, and people in an occupied territory have their rights. Occupying oppressors have to leave.

I would also stress that these atrocities must not merely be regarded as human rights violations. They *are* human rights violations, no doubt, but the issue is beyond that and merits focus of every forum. These agonising atrocities are war crimes. Until the occupation ends, the state of war shall continue to exist. The incessant occupation qualifies these atrocities as war crimes. Of course crimes against humanity can be committed even in the times of peace. But, as I said before, my position is that this is a case of occupation, and it tells us that a state of war exists in Kashmir.

Since, an evident state of war exists; these atrocities ought to be termed as war crimes. The people who are supportive of the Kashmir cause should, at least in academia, highlight that Kashmir is not only an issue of human rights violations, rather these are war crimes, and criminal law should be applied to the oppressor as far as the International Committee of the Red Cross is concerned.

I acknowledge that the ICRC has been making efforts for the last 70 years. Yet, what we expect from the ICRC is a clear acknowledgement and recognition of the fact that this is an international conflict. The aspect of occupation has not been stressed the way it should have been.

Since Kashmir is occupied and occupation means war, this conflict qualifies as an International Armed Conflict, and must be treated as so.

Struggle for Right to Self-Determination and War Crimes in IOK

Ambassador Ashraf Qazi[4]

I confess that I am not an international lawyer, or a lawyer of any kind, but I have been a career diplomat, and of course, Kashmir has been atop the foreign policy agenda of Pakistan. Therefore, we have always tried to familiarize ourselves with the basic legal aspects of the dispute. And apart from the legal aspects, there are the diplomatic aspects, and then, there the extra diplomatic aspects that need to be considered when all else fails in the UN Security Council.

The issue is listed on the agenda as the India-Pakistan question. This is in accordance with the India Independence Act 1947, which stated that the princely states of British India would accede to either India or Pakistan in accordance with the wishes of the majority of their people, even when the rulers who may be of a different faith, make a decision without regarding the majority opinion.

The UNSC resolution 39 of 20th January, 1948 called for UN administered plebiscite to be held in Jammu and Kashmir for the people to decide whether they wished to join India

[4]Ambassador Ashraf Qazi is former diplomat. He has served in the US and many other regions as Ambassador of Pakistan

or Pakistan. India accepted the resolution and Jawaharlal Nehru conceded if the vote went against India, though he would bitterly regret it, he would accept it.

India immediately began complicating the work of the UN commission for India and Pakistan, which was set up to organize the UN-administered plebiscite. India launched genocide in Jammu to convert it from a 61% Muslim majority region to a Muslim minority region. More than 300,000 Muslims were killed. These figures may or may not be exact but they showed the magnitude and an even greater number expelled into Azad Jammu and Pakistan.

When Pakistan joined the US-led security to secure itself against what it saw as Indian threats, Nehru used it as an excuse to withdraw Indian support from the UN resolutions, and India refused to demilitarize the region. The UNSC resolutions for Jammu and Kashmir were taken under Chapter VI of the UN charter, which is concerned with the pacific settlement of disputes rather than under Chapter VII, which is concerned with action with respect to threats to the breaches of the peace and acts of aggression. It is commonly mistaken that UN resolutions under Chapter VII are obligatory while under Chapter VI are only advisory; this is utterly wrong. Either chapter has the same legal status and is obligatory. The only difference is that under Chapter VII, the resolutions are enforceable, according to some legal experts. The designation of the UN resolutions as under Chapter VI or VII is a much later development than when the first resolutions were adopted.

Moreover, under Article 99 of the UN Charter, the UN secretary general, if he thinks the situation threatens the peace in a specific region, can refer the matter to the UNSC for urgent consideration. There have been, at least, three Indo-Pak wars over this issue. And since August 5, 2019, India has escalated both – its war-like rhetoric against Pakistan, and violence across the Line of Control.

The UN secretary general has more than ever an obligation to take these developments into consideration, and refer the matter to the UNSC under Article 99 for immediate consideration with reference to all the previous UN resolutions on Jammu and Kashmir which remain valid, in other words: *de facto*. If not, then the UNSC resolutions on Jammu and Kashmir can take on some of the character of Chapter VII resolutions in the event the UNSG sees the urgency of the matter according to UNSC Resolution 122 of 1957.

The UN refuses to recognize the alleged accession of Jammu and Kashmir to India in violation of existing UN resolutions. In other words, India might seek to create facts in Indian-occupied Kashmir, but it cannot create international law for Jammu and Kashmir, which is not an Indian territory and, accordingly, beyond the writ of the Indian Constitution as per the Article 370, which has now been scrapped.

The introduction of draconian laws in IOK, the massive violation of human rights including several massacres, and the impunity under Armed Forces' Special Powers Act 1990 has allowed Indian perpetrators carry on with their atrocities. And now, another lockdown has been imposed due to COVID-19, which is not for the protection of the people's health, but for the repression and elimination of the vast majority of the people of the valley who refuse to consider themselves as Indians. India is determined to eliminate them as they are an obstacle to the absorption of Kashmir into India.

The United Nations General Assembly in its Resolution 3314 in 1974 and then again in 1982 recognized the right of oppressed people to wage struggle, including *armed struggle,* but forcibly usurped the right to self-determination.

The resolutions also recognize the right of the oppressed to solicit assistance, including armed assistance from abroad, to carry on their legitimate struggle against oppression and the forcible denial of their legitimate and recognized rights while condemning aggression in all its forms. These resolutions specifically include armed struggle on behalf of recognized international rights, including the right of self-determination.

Since 9/11 the so-called war on terror waged by the US and its allies, there have been attempts by international lawyers from these countries to deny the right of armed struggle under any circumstances, including the right of self-determination. However, the UN has never recognized Kashmir having acceded to India. Accordingly, denial of the unacknowledged right of armed struggle on behalf of the right to self-determination cannot be rescinded in any circumstance.

So, where do we go from here?

On August 5, 2019, Indian Prime Minister Narendra Modi decided to eliminate the already hollowed out special status of occupied Kashmir under the Indian Constitution, and to eliminate it as a political entity, by making it a union (federal) territory.

This has hugely compounded India's defiance of international law. India is relying on its supposed great power status which, in its view, entitles it to make international law for others and not to be bound itself by the law. Six days later, on August 11, 2019, Genocide Watch issued a Genocide Alert regarding the situation in IOK, with reference to the Genocide Convention on the Prevention and Punishment of the Crime of Genocide in 1948.

In Article 2 of the Genocide Convention, Genocide is defined as "*any of the following acts committed with the intent to destroy, in whole or in part, a national ethnic, racial, or religious group as such and it includes killing members of the group causing serious bodily or mental harm to members of the group deliberately inflicting on the group conditions of life calculated to bring about its physical destruction in whole or in part imposing measures intended to prevent births within the group forcibly, transferring children of the group to another group*".

The Genocide Watch and Genocide Alert listed 10 stages of the genocidal process in IOK as being far advanced, and these include a number of categories.

The first one is classification: Hindu and Sikh Indian army versus Muslim civilians, in other words, us versus them. Muslim names on their ID cards, language, dress, mosques etc.

Hindu Pandits were economically dominant until 1990 and later the ruling Bharatiya Janta Party (BJP) reasserted Hindu power through dehumanization. Muslims are called terrorists, criminals, separatist, insurgents etc.

While there are 600,000 occupying troops besides paramilitaries and police in the region, the BJP and its supporters incite anti-Muslim hatred through social media by spreading falsehoods. Muslims were under severe movement restrictions, well before the novel coronavirus. They are persecuted, subjected to arrest, tortured, and raped, and murderously exterminated.

A genocidal massacre has been taking place since 1990. There have been countless massacres of Muslims since partition.

In view of the above, the Genocide Watch called upon the UN and its members to warn India against genocide. It is important because we hardly see the word 'genocide' in Pakistani statements. Yes, in the beginning there was much mention of it and then reportedly, some of the UN's senior officials pleaded to avoid the use of such language since it is provocative and sought to "ameliorate" the situation by avoiding such terms. But under international law, Genocide Watch, and in accordance with the Genocide Convention, what India did proved to be tantamount to progressive genocide a year later.

It is time for the Genocide Watch to upgrade its Genocide Alert to a Genocide Warning, which if not heeded by India or the international community will lead to the final stage of the genocide process, which is known as a Genocide Emergency.

Pakistan's response has so far been restricted to diplomacy and lawfare. It has achieved fewer successes, and more setbacks. Pakistan's efforts need to be intensified and improved. It is a brutal reality that it will never be sufficient to elicit international pressure on India, so much so that its reverses its policy of progressive genocide in IOK, and threats against Azad Jammu and Pakistan.

While I appreciate Pakistan's support, it has been unable to make a decisive difference to Kashmir's plight.

An alliance has been formed in Indian-occupied Kashmir, which calls for a reversal of the New Delhi's unilateral decision on August 5. Many of these leaders had earlier said that they had learnt a lesson, and realised they made a blunder by trusting India that it would abide by Kashmir's special status. And now, they are left not with three options of India, Pakistan or *Azadi* (freedom) but only two: *Azadi* or Pakistan.

If Pakistan withdraws support, the Kashmir struggle will still sustain but will be hugely compromised. And it could well be overwhelmed by India's progressive policy of genocide, just because of the sheer momentum of the size of India versus the resistance in IOK. If Pakistan chooses in such a circumstance to be a passive witness to this massive atrocity, having already lost its majority in 1971, there will be a real danger of the country of losing all its meaning. The consequences, to put it very mildly, will be unmanageable. Despite all the diplomacy and lawfare, India cannot be made to reverse its policy because the international community is simply not ready to do so for a number of reasons: power politics, economic factors, and of course Pakistan's image. These things affect Pakistan's arguments on Kashmir.

Even though they are correct in terms of law , Pakistan is in a dilemma: be a passive witness or finding some kind of out-of-the-box diplomatic solution.

In my view, Pakistan should consider a two-track policy towards Kashmir. It should involve the search for a peaceful settlement, a principled compromised settlement, which was attempted through backchannels a few years ago, though controversial in Pakistan. Many supported it as the only possible option, while others called it an outright betrayal of the cause.

But then of course, we need to recognize the reality that there can never be a zero-sum solution to the problem such that Pakistan wins and India loses, or vice versa. This is not possible because it will not be consistent in maintaining peace and the stability in the region. One has to regard the fact that the two countries do have a significant deterrent capacity, making zero-sum solutions impossible. Positive solutions are the only way forward.

The problem now is that Narendra Modi sees himself as so powerful that he is not willing to consider any kind of compromise and therefore, Pakistan is left with no option but to follow a two-track policy. The first track should seek a dialogue with India for improvement in the human rights situation and a gradual incremental cumulative progress towards a principled compromise settlement, which is acceptable primarily to the people of Kashmir, and also then, the peoples of Pakistan and India. The likelihood of this track succeeding today is extremely low because of Modi and the BJP's hardline. It was not such when the Indian National Congress was in power.

In India, though there is opposition to the violation of human rights, but little recognition of political rights of Kashmiris. The denial and violation of human rights is directly derived from the denial of political rights. If you address the political rights, you will set the scene for a major improvement in human rights. This is what India refuses to discuss. Therefore, there is no hope of an improvement in the human rights situation in Kashmir, and it is remorseful that inevitably, the progress towards genocide will not cease, let alone, be reversed.

Thus, the second track, followed simultaneously with the first track, is: To tell the world, credibly, that Pakistan is seeking a peaceful settlement. We are willing to go out of our way, and walk the extra mile. But, if we are snubbed, and India continues its violations, Pakistan will be forced to see it as an existential threat to it, and left with no option but to do all it can to stop India.

We will have to convey, with our peace initiatives, Pakistan's peaceful nature and sincerity. We must improve our image, but at the same time our warnings need to credible. We must convey that if India continues to ignore Pakistan's initiatives towards a genuine societal solution, then Pakistan *will* go out of its way to stop that no matter what the cost may be.

This is the only way to prevent genocide and prevent war between India and Pakistan. If the international community realises the credibility of this warning, the pressure on India would mount and increase to the point where India could be forced to take a second look at its policies, with respect to not only its August 5 decision, but also a final settlement, a compromise-settlement, acceptable to all three parties. Should we be able to reach such a compromised settlement that would be legally possible, we have to make it politically possible, too. A new UNSC resolution acceptable to all three parties – Kashmir, Pakistan, and India – embodying such a settlement must be unanimously adopted then. This will open wider avenues for Pakistan-India relationships. Having championed the rights of the people, there are no perfect solutions; there are no risk-free solutions; there are no cost-free solutions; but if we pretend to be going for an absolute solution, an absolute victory over India, then in reality, we will be going for nothing. And we will be in a sense seen by our brothers as totally misleading them and many of them are already saying Pakistan has given up the struggle.

Gross Human Rights Abuse in Indian-occupied Kashmir and Silence of the International Community

Dr Ghulam Nabi Fai[5]

I would like to remind everybody that we are mindful that there have been hundreds of webinars within the past few months, but these brought no change to the situation. So, the very first question arises: why do we need to have one more and what justifies holding another?

Yes, it is true that these webinars did not produce any tangible results on the ground but it is also true that not organizing these virtual summits will have the most damaging, devastating, and painful impact on the situation in IOK.

If we fail to have a discussion, it is going to strengthen the impression created by Narendra Modi and his administration that conflict has no life left in it. It is also going to strengthen the impression that the exertion of Indian military might have settled the matters in Kashmir, and that the atrocities committed by Indian army have compelled the people of to accept Indian occupation.

Ladies and gentlemen, we know that this impression is absolutely false, and that is why it is important that we must erase that impression. Thereby, I have to give the description of the situation in, but please allow me to say just a few words before that, about the ground reality.

[5] Dr Ghulam Nabi Fai is global Kashmiri diaspora leader and secretary general of US-based World Kashmir Awareness Forum

There was a survey conducted by the London-based Chatham House, released by the BBC on May 27, 2010. It was a long questionnaire on what a majority of Kashmiris want, and that is *Azadi (freedom).*

When India came to know about the findings, it got frustrated. And the immediate reaction from India when people demand freedom is that it says they do not know what they are talking about.

The catch phrase of the freedom struggle on the streets does not mean autonomy. Let me also be clear here with the fullest possible consciousness, *Azadi* does not mean General Pervez Musharraf's four-point formula. *Azadi* does not mean backdoor diplomacy of which Kashmiris are not a part of.

I will quote Arundhati Roy, one of the most recognizable Indian human rights activists. When asked on October 3, 2019, what do the people want, she said, and I quote, "The people of Kashmir have been saying it for the last 70 years; the people of Kashmir have been saying it with their blood; the people want the right to self-determination." She reiterated, "They want the right to self-determination."

For the people of Kashmir, more than 100,000 of their lives sacrificed are not for backdoor diplomacy; the situation is alarming and terrifying. They say that there has been an Indian military crackdown for the last one year, which is absolutely false. The clampdown is continuing for the last 29 years. It began on the unfortunate night of February 23, 1991 in Kunan-Poshpora, twin villages in northern Kashmir. More than 100 of our sisters were raped by the occupying army.

These lockdowns during COVID-19 may be unique to the world but not for Kashmiris.

The Indian army is using pellet guns on peaceful processions.

What is going on in Kashmir? If you're a journalist, you can write anything you want to write, but you cannot write what the Indian army is doing. If you do, you will have to face the consequences. There are hundreds of examples, I will give you just one: Asif Sultan. His articles appeared not only in India but in the international press. What was his crime? He committed the same crime committed by Yashwant Sinha. He was the BJP foreign minister, when he said, and I quote, "India, you are making one after another mistake…"

This is exactly what Asif Sultan said, "India, you are making one after another mistake." He was picked up and detained under Unlawful Activity Prevention Act. Anybody picked up under this can be declared as a terrorist. This law violates four articles of Universal Declaration of Human Rights, i.e. Article 7, 9, 10, and 11. It also violates five articles of the International Covenant on Civil and Political Rights: Article 6, 7, 19, 21, and 22.

People have no access to the internet. Doctors are unable to treat their patients. They are unable to consult anyone outside Kashmir. It's a matter of life and death.

Another thing that poses an existential threat to Kashmiris is the domicile law. No foreigner can settle in IOK and no foreigner can buy land. One must have a domicile certificate if one wants to settle here, have a job or buy property here.

India is changing the demography because it knows that the existing populace in Kashmir is not going to vote for India.

Multiple resolutions say that a unilateral action cannot be taken to change the status of a disputed state. This begs the very question: why is the international community silent?

Antonio Guterres, the secretary general of the United Nations, just three days later, on August 8, 2019, came to our support. He gave us hope. He is, after all, the custodian of human rights. He reiterated that the Kashmir issue is to be resolved according to the UN Charter, and under the applicable UNSC resolutions.

When India imposed a ban on internet, Narendra Modi said it was to stop terrorism. The UN special rapporteur on freedom of expression said Kashmir must have internet to stop disinformation, protect civil liberties and hold the authorities to account. India is committing countless human rights violations under the leadership of "butcher of Gujarat."

Narendra Modi responded that no one should intervene in India's "internal affairs.". Six hundred and fifty members of the European Parliament, and five congressional hearings and the briefings in Washington DC condemned the violations.

Six internationally recognized NGOs, including the Amnesty International, Geneva-based International Commission of Jurisdiction (ICJ), Paris-based International Federation of Human Rights, and Manila-based South Asian Community on Human Rights, made a joint statement that the people of Kashmir have all the right to express their opinion, and called for the release of political prisoners.

On August 5, 17 UN reports were released, which not only condemned the human rights violations but said India failed to fulfull its promise to improve the human rights situation. But, unfortunately, they failed to recognize it was their responsibility to intervene in the matter.

The New York Times in one of its articles remarked: '*Paradise does not exist anymore.*' It said, *"India has made hell for the people of Kashmir."*

When Narendra Modi boasted that India is the largest democracy in the world, *The Huffington Post* wrote: *"Indian democracy is dead."*

There is no mercy in Kashmir. Nine hundred thousand Indian military personnel have made it the largest military zone in the world.

Yes, it is true that these voices are there. But, they have yet to translate their understanding into tangible actions. The UN high commissioner on human rights has an important post. She has been the elected president of Chile for 10 years. She was recommended to send a fact-finding mission to India. India, as expected, said no.

One may wonder, since India claims to be the largest democracy, how on earth could India violate all these international laws?

India knows that it is one of the largest economies in the world. It knows the world is dealing with COVID-19, and world powers may not pay attention to the situation in IOK. And unfortunately, the world powers have always remained silent.

But, the world powers do not know that their silence, their inefficiency, and their passivity has given a sense of total impunity to the Indian army. Otherwise, how could one justify that a person, no less important than Donald Trump, offering his office for mediation but to no avail?

India said no and Donald Trump took the 'no' of India as an answer. There could be many reasons for America's passivity. The US has signed commercial contracts worth billions of dollars with India. It also wants India to act as a shield against the rise of China. Thereby, all universal values and international norms have become victim to commercial interests.

That's why it is your responsibility and it is my responsibility, and it is our collective responsibility to knock at the door of every single member of the United Nations, and tell them two things: You accepted the right to self-determination of the people of Kashmir through the UNSC Resolution 47, which was adopted on April 21, 1948, written under the instructions of President Harry Truman by US ambassador to UN Warren Austin, and tell them that Kashmir is the only region in the world that shares borders with three nuclear powers of the world.

India and Pakistan are on the brink of a nuclear confrontation, the bone of contention, the source of friction and the underlying cause of this tension is nothing but the issue that the UN must intervene in. World powers must come out of slumber to resolve the issues not only for the sake of IOK, but also for the sake of South Asia, where 1.5 billion people reside.

I tell the leadership of Pakistan that we understand the compulsions and pressures you are in. In any case, do not pursue the option of "autonomy." Please, if you cannot help us, let the people of Kashmir be left alone, they will handle it.

On August 13, 2020, a special curfew imposed by New Delhi for two days – 14 and 15. They had reports that the people were going to celebrate 15th August as a Black Day. India knows they have been able to arrest and kill more than 100,000 people, disappear more than 10,000 and tortured many more. Chinese ambassador Zhang Kali mentioned correctly: it's a routine here. They have not been able to win over the hearts and minds of the people.

Ramifications of Military Occupation in IOK

Justice Ali Nawaz Chowhan[6]

As illustrated by my fellows, all the United Nations resolutions have always been overlooked. We see that the human rights violations go on without any stop. One wonders, what would be the ramifications of a prolonged stay of India's occupying forces?

Legally speaking, this has no impact and we have seen in the case of the independence movement of all nations, including that of the subcontinent, a hundred years or so of

[6] Justice Chowhan is former Judge at Hague and Chief Justice of Gambia. He is presently Honorary Chairman LFK

'occupation' by a colonial power, made no difference. And when we stood for our independence, we won prescriptive rights. There is no such thing as prescriptive rights in the international law because this occupation is a usurp and there are doctrines to the effect that whatever changes they may be making, whatever they may be doing, will have no consequence. But, what are the practical consequences? We see on one hand, people are suffering, the human rights are being violated, and war crimes are being committed with impunity, and we find no remedy at hand, unless we craft one to stop the war crimes.

Under Article 99 of the UN, the secretary general is supposed to take a notice of these atrocities. The high commissioner in Geneva is also supposed to pay attention. Yet, we find that there is complete silence. At the hands of India's 900,000 soldiers, the people of Kashmir are being subjected to crimes, which you could only compare with holocaust, or the ones committed in Rwanda, or by the Serbs in the former Yugoslavia and so on and so forth. But they were held accountable for the ethnic cleansing, genocide and destruction of property and religious sites.

When the big powers have an interest, of course, they will create institutions and conduct trials. The magnitude, the quantum of wrongs being committed by India is no less than some of the examples that I have quoted. I'm not going to repeat the history and the UN resolutions, which my colleagues have already explained in detail but rather discuss how to go about it now.

There are two aspects: one relates to human rights and violation of human rights with impunity, while the other is of territorial dispute between the two states of India and Pakistan.

As far as the territorial dispute is concerned, well the states are already engaged. The states should go ahead with whatever remedies are available, whether political or otherwise. Because there is a commitment as well that the matters are to be resolved in a peaceful manner.

This happened subsequently because of the war and because of the declarations between Pakistan and India. Then the present matter, where we can go forward against India is the human rights issue. Now this human rights aspect is, of course, subject to further investigation. It would be good if Pakistan went against India since it has *locus standi*. If Gambia can go against Myanmar in the International Court of Justice, why not Pakistan against India?

I would urge the government of Pakistan and our prime minister, who wants to resolve this issue, to go ahead with it.

But, if not, we can choose other avenues as ambassador Jehangir Qazi has said, as citizens of Pakistan, brothers of Kashmiris, all of us can join hands.

We can take this issue to the National Institution of Human Rights (NIHR). I've been a chairman of one of such institutions, and know their strength. They are independent.

All the members of what they call as the gallery, if we make them aware and keep them aware of all the atrocities, we will have a great public world opinion. In that case, India will have to hide its face and that will be one of the greatest pressures we can put on India without getting into politics.

Then there are matters we can take to the UN. Under Article 99, Islamabad can speak about the violations of human rights and urge the secretary general to take cognizance, like a *suo moto* notice. Why can't that be done?

The idea is to agitate the issue to a certain extent that India starts hearing and behaving.

Facts should be brought to the notice of the international community. India already is on a sticky wicket and is trying to win diplomatic support. Unfortunately, many Muslim countries are also trying, in a passive way, to support India by not objecting to the annexation of a territory, which is absolutely disputed and consists of Muslims. The division of India took place on the basis of the principle that Muslim-majority regions will go to Pakistan but to no avail.

I must tell you that a book has been written by one of our representatives in the United Nations, Sir Zafarullah Khan, who has spoken of the agony of Pakistan and given us a glimpse of the background of conspiracies of Jawaharlal Nehru and Lord Mountbatten, and how the great powers were involved ultimately because of their closeness and common grounds.

Yet, we have a great game, and in that great game there are common interests of great nations and they don't bother whether it is Palestine or Kashmir.

Yes, we hear of human rights, of actions against genocide, conventions on war crimes, genocide, and civil and political rights, and civil and economic rights and so on. But practically, when it comes to the involvement of world powers, interest is supreme. They just don't let it go. But they do respect public opinion, i.e. the Black Lives Matter movement.

Let us not also forget that the Blacks fought for their rights for decades. I don't mean that this should last also for many years. Over 70 years have already passed. But we must find out alternate ways to raise human rights issues and that is my point.

This may bring some relief to the suffering people of who deserve all the sympathy, and all the support. We don't want things to go be forgotten like the 1947 Jammu massacre.

Now, they want to change the demographics, and that itself, falls under ethnic cleansing, which is a war crime. We ask the UNSC to constitute a tribunal for war crimes to see what India has done, and investigate.

Of course, in the case of Afghanistan, the superpower will not allow that to happen. But in the case of Kashmir, we may go forward. But how do we keep the pressure on this is important.

The resolutions make no difference, because they have already become a part of books and record. We have to discover new methods to come out of it and then go forward with the innovation and new ideas to put India to shame, internationally.

Question and Answer Session

Both India and Pakistan are not party to Additional Protocol I of Geneva Convention, which legitimises the war of liberation based on the right to self-determination, what would be the situation on this?

Dr Muhammad Mushtaq:

Neither Pakistan nor India is party to this protocol. The point is -- it is necessary for one to be a party to a treaty, for the application of the treaty on that state. However, it is also a fact that sometimes, there are parallel rules of customary nature, which are found in state practice, and they are also found in some treaty. So, Customary Law and the treaty become synonymous as well as analogous. And, of course, in that case Customary Law binds all states.

Thus, the armed liberation struggle of Kashmir has become an International Armed Conflict; it has become part of Customary International Law (CIL).

Scholars around the globe agree on this. Kashmir's armed struggle for liberation is not only an international conflict but also a part of Customary Law; and as part of Customary Law, it is applicable to all states.

What is the legal remedy available to approach UN? Where can we build the narrative of a distinction between terrorism and liberation movement?

Dr Muhammad Mushtaq:

Instead of just talking about human rights violations, we should make a case for considering these atrocities as war crimes. Kashmir is under occupation, which is illegal. Occupation constitutes a state of war. That is why these atrocities ought to be considered as war crimes, not just human rights violations.

Prior to the adoption of the Kellogg–Briand Pact of Paris in 1928 , one could talk about occupation as one of the means for acquiring title to a territory. However, since that particular treaty has been adopted, international law has considered occupation and annexation as illegal.

Now, our case is -- the state of Jammu Kashmir was occupied; part of it was liberated later but the rest remains occupied. And since, it is occupied and it is in a state of constant war, it is facing an International Armed Conflict. The atrocities committed here are not just violations of human rights' laws but war crimes.

Although, neither Pakistan nor India is party to the Rome Statute, there are three ways to bring the case to the International Criminal Court:

1. A state party refers the case to the ICC. Of course, this option is not available.

2. The UNSC, actin, under Chapter VII of the UN Charter, refers the case to the ICC. This option is also unlikely to materialise.

Then, there is a third option: the prosecutor of the ICC, based on reports available with the office, can bring the issue before the ICC and the pre-trial chamber will look into it to see if there are enough grounds for moving ahead. The ICC can take up the case this way.

So, why not try this way; why not bring all these cases and all the evidence and reports on atrocities of various kinds committed by the Indian troops in Kashmir?

We bring them in the form of petitions, of course, supported by evidence to the office of the prosecutor. And, we could make a move for this purpose supported by various actors and bring it to the limelight and compel the prosecutor's office to make a case. Now, it is true that a case in the ICC takes a long time, and costs extravagantly; one has to consider many options.

Explain the role of the International Committee of the Red Cross (ICRC) in the Kashmir conflict. It does not enter IOK and observe on-the-ground situation there.

Dr Muhammad Mushtaq:

As far as the ICRC's role is concerned, the ICRC in its working modality is a bit different; it works with the consent of the parties to the conflict.

It seeks access. Of course, it cites many provisions of the Geneva Conventions, which make it obligatory on these parties to allow access to the ICRC. But, it depends on the bill of consent of the particular party. Even if a state refuses to give access to the ICRC, it has many ways to build pressure.

Meanwhile, the head office of the ICRC for South Asia is in New Delhi. The entire region is looked after by the New Delhi office of the ICRC, except Pakistan.

India does have influence over the people working there. Even if the ICRC officially does not acknowledge this, there is no denying this fact. This may be one of the many possible reasons for ICRC's dormancy.

But again, I should come back to my initial point that we have to present our case in a different manner. Instead of talking about whether or not the conflict has reached the threshold of international conflict, we should make up a case that this has been an International Armed Conflict since the beginning. It has been an International Armed Conflict throughout.

Let us make our case this way; let us convince the ICRC as well that it has a mandate and it has an obligation, which it must fulfil under the Geneva Conventions and under its own statute.

Can the Azad Jammu and Kashmir Assembly pass a resolution that we are within our rights to liberate the Indian-occupied territory through armed struggle?

Dr Muhammad Mushtaq:

Under the international law perspective, from the beginning, the idea has been that Azad Kashmir and its government should be at the forefront, and kind of a base camp for valley's liberation struggle.

Unfortunately, for various reasons, political and other, this could not be done. But, it is never too late. We have to reconsider this policy.

Policymakers have to reconsider their position. The Azad Jammu and Kashmir government should lead and Pakistan should support it. For example, when France was occupied during World War I, a government in exile was formed and it was supported by the allied forces during WWII, and special provisions were included in the Geneva Conventions, about the definition of "combatants" and "prisoners of war" – Article Six and Article Four in the third Geneva Convention where these people were given the status of combatants and when captured, the status of prisoners of war.

Why not use those provisions? Why not give this particular status to the freedom fighters of Kashmir? The Azad Jammu and Kashmir government should come to the forefront. It should take the leading role. It should present the case to the world, and Pakistan should support it.

As far as the reference to Article 257 of Pakistan Constitution is concerned, the reference was given by respected ambassador Qazi.

With all due respect, I would say that Article 257 of the Pakistan's Constitution does not allow room for the third option.

Let me read the provisions of this Article 257. I quote, "*When the people of the state of Jammu and Kashmir decide to accede to Pakistan, the relationship between Pakistan and the State shall be determined in accordance with the wishes of the people of their state.*"

It simply describes what kind of relationship will be there... what powers will stay with the central and the federal government... what powers will be given to the newly acceded province, after accession to Pakistan; after the people of the state of Jammu and Kashmir accede to Pakistan.

This is about post-existing situation, if and when the people of the state of Jammu and Kashmir accede to Pakistan. Thence, the future constitutional setup would be decided in accordance with the wishes of the people. How much of autonomy will be given, what powers should be given to them, what powers should be retained by the federation, all will be decided according to the will of the people.

Session II

Kashmir's Liberation Movement for Right to Self-Determination

Dr. Niaz Shah[7]

Is the Kashmiri liberation movement for the right to self-determination by indigenous rebel groups against occupying forces in Indian-occupied Kashmir (IOK) legal under international law? What are the similarities and differences between Islamic and international humanitarian laws?

As a human rights lawyer, I am looking at these questions from the legal perspective.

I think the second part of the question is slightly misconceived; the right to self-determination is not really a part of international humanitarian law.

As we shall see later in my brief discussion that emanates from the UN Charter. I shall briefly talk about the right to self-determination under international law. I have also noted some options for Kashmiris regarding how they can go about the realization of their right.

In international law, the right to self-determination is well established and starts from the UN Charter.

The purpose of the United Nations is *to develop friendly relations among nations, based on respect for the principle of equal rights and self-determination of peoples; and to take other appropriate measures to strengthen universal peace.*

[7] Niaz A. Shah is barrister and professor in law. He is author of several book including Islam and the law of armed conflict. He is one of the general editors of journals of international humanitarian legal studies. He also worked as a protection assistant for UNHCR and remain consultant of UNICEF. He is currently working on research project Application of International Human rights law in Muslims states.

Now, when you look at this first article, you find that universal peace is tied to respect for equal rights and self-determination. This, indeed, is the foundational article in the UN Charter because it sets out the purpose for the existence of the UN. If we go further in the UN Charter, in Article 55 again, the same language is used to say that with the view to *"create the condition of stability and well-being, which are necessary for peaceful and friendly relations among nations based on respect for the principle of equal rights and self-determination of the peoples".*

Thus, international peace and security are linked to the right to self-determination.

The main function of the UN is to restore international peace and security and to resolve disputes, peacefully. Now, it's also mentioned in the Universal Declaration of Human Rights.

The binding two treaties covered in the International Covenants of 1966 of the UN have a common article, which deals with self-determination.

This common article of the ICCPR, and its sister covenant – International Covenant on Economic Social and Cultural Rights – put the right to self-determination above and before every other article in the structure and the composition of these two covenants.

Paragraph one of Common Article 1 of the International Covenant on Civil and Political Rights states that all people have the right of self-determination.

It explains that by virtue of their right, they can freely determine their political status and pursue their economic, social and cultural development. Paragraph 3 of the common article is even more crucial, because it imposes certain positive obligations on states (parties). It says *the state-parties to the present covenant including those having responsibility for the administration of non-self-governing interest territories shall promote the realization of the right to self-determination.*

The language here is important: "*Shall promote the realization of the right of self-determination.*" To respect promotion is one obligation and to show respect is another. There is a major difference between the two.

"Respect" here would really require positive actions on the part of state parties to take measures to respect that right of self-determination. The International Covenant on Civil and Political Rights has 173 parties, which include India and Pakistan.

When India, in April 1979, acceded to this covenant, it entered a declaration. India is trying to put its own interpretation to this article, which imposes positive obligation. India claims that the right to self-determination appearing in this article applies only to the people under foreign domination. But if you look and compare this language with the clear language of the Common Article 1, there is a clear mismatch.

What India is trying here is basically to impose an interpretation which clearly goes against the spirit, purpose, and objective of the two treaties. This is a strategic move. The claim Kashmir is an integral part and is not occupied or dominated by a foreign power allows India to evade from these aforementioned obligations, according to India's propaganda. Thereby, India is imposing and proposing that Kashmiris don't have the right to self-determination.

Sovereign states have their own right to make declarations, but that doesn't mean they cannot be questioned under international law, and thus, India's acts are questionable.

There are several judgments of the International Court of Justice, which clearly establish that the right to self-determination has a broad scope. In the case of East Timor, Portugal versus Australia, 1995 judgment, just by looking at the bare and clear language, one could see that it is well established.

The population living in any zone should have a territory, common culture, religion, and location so I don't see any difficulty in establishing that they meet the requirement of the definition of people.

Now, the question is: how they can realize their right to determine their future? The first would be the democratic method. India tried to control the results of such a method forcefully, which were rejected by the Kashmiris.

Since the status of Kashmir is disputed, there are no two views looking at a number of strings of Security Council resolutions, the inherent spirit and the mechanism of the charter in human rights law is to resolve disputes peacefully. That is the spirit reflected in the UN Security Council resolutions on Kashmir. Therefore, the best way forward is to hold a free and fair plebiscite in accordance with the UN Security Council (UNSC) resolutions.

India, being a member of the United Nations, has an obligation under the UN Charter and needs to respect and promote the right of self-determination. All the member states need to promote and respect the right of self-determination under the charter, and more specifically, under the UNSC resolutions.

India is a state party to the International Covenant in Civil and Political Rights (ICCPR). And under Article 1 of the ICCPR, it is required to promote the right to self-determination and respect it. And as I said before, this would require positive measures. So, when you tie these threads together – the Security Council, the UN Charter, and the International Human Rights Law (IHRL), the burden heavily falls on India as a UN member state and a state party to take positive measures and to go for the suggested method, democratically.

Another option is for individuals, to take cases to the Human Rights Committee under the ICCPR. But, India is not party to the first Optional Protocol, so this option is not available in general. The Human Rights Committee tends to say that the right to self-determination belongs to people, and not individuals. This position is heavily criticized by academics and experts.

Hence, the option of the armed struggle appears to be last resort. Although, the spirit of the UN Charter is to resolve disputes peacefully and human rights law is also about peace, what happens in reality is that people wait for decades, give peace a chance but to no avail. Hence, they're faced with a dilemma: give up their right to self-determination and live as oppressed and subjugated people, or start an armed resistance.

The case of Kashmir seems to fall in this category. Kashmiris have waited far too long, yet the dispute is not resolved. It was 1948 when the Indian ambassador first reported the matter to the UNSC. And since then, it is dormant there. For how long does one wait for peaceful means to produce results before turning to armed struggle? That is the real question here.

Pakistan Diplomacy Post-annexation

Ambassador Abdul Basit[8]

Dr. Niaz has had a very interesting, informative, educative articulation of the legal aspect of the right to self-determination. At least, I learned a lot today.

Now, the question that I would try to address here is to explore any space for diplomacy to resolve this long-standing issue after India's unconstitutional and illegal action, which it took on August 5, 2019.

We all know that since the 1972 Simla Agreement, India has been insisting that this dispute between India and Pakistan is bilateral in nature. India has been insisting that since Pakistan has agreed to talk bilaterally with India, it is now between Pakistan and India to resolve this issue through peaceful means and through dialogue.

But, as Dr. Niaz Shah very rightly pointed out, even after more than almost 50 years, the bilateral engagement between Pakistan and India has not produced any result as far as Jammu and Kashmir is concerned.

We have been talking to each other but, unfortunately, we have always found India prevaricating from the dispute itself. It has been trying to buy time to engage Pakistan on peripheral issues and does not come to the core dispute. Though at one point of time between 2004 and 2007 there was some back channel diplomacy going on between the two countries, but even in that era India gradually diverted from Kashmir to other issues, particularly the issues related to terrorism.

---

[8] Abdul Basit, a retired Pakistani diplomat who served as a former High Commissioner of Pakistan to India in New Delhi. He was also appointed as Ambassador to Germany. During his career he was posted at Moscow, New York, sanna and London.

After 9/11 in particular, India has been trying to portray the entire Kashmir struggle as terrorism, supported and abetted by Pakistan. And after 2008, when some unknown people conspired in Mumbai attacks, though the trial is still on in Pakistan, India has shown no desire or readiness to talk on Kashmir.

I have been part of many meetings with India on this particular issue and I can say from my own experience that there is simply no desire on the part of India to discuss Kashmir in a meaningful, result-oriented manner.

Back in 2014, when elections were being held in India, the BJP manifesto talked about revoking Article 370 of the Indian Constitution and stripping the occupied Jammu and Kashmir of its special status. When it happened on August 5, at least I was not surprised or shocked, since this was going to happen sooner or later.

If you ask me of international intervention, I do not see it happening soon because, fortunately or unfortunately, the international community seems to be indifferent to what is happening or what India has done to Jammu and Kashmir.

The world as a whole is not keen to put pressure on India, even on improving human rights situation on the ground, like revoking draconian laws such as such as Armed Force Special Powers Act (AFSPA), Public Safety Act (PSA), and the Disturbed Areas Act (DDA).

If you look at the mainland India, civil societies mostly subscribe to the official viewpoint of India that the Kashmir struggle is mostly about terrorism.

Even in occupied Kashmir itself, while the majority of Kashmiris are struggling for their right to determination, one may find voices who do accept occupied Kashmir as part of India. Therefore, in terms of diplomacy, frankly speaking, I am not very optimistic. Because, there is neither pressure on India from within nor from abroad regarding Kashmir, for a variety of reasons.

India is seen by the world as a rising economy. Though it has shrunk during the last six months, India is a huge market for international powers. There are commercial interests, and economic interests involved here. The global dynamics are also changing.

India has become a strategic partner of the United States and the West. So, there are strong reasons as to why the international community is largely quiet on the issue of Jammu and Kashmir.

Yes, we do hear voices, here and there sometimes, about human rights. The UN human rights commissioner talks about it. But the report on human rights issued in June 2018 is not adopted by the UN Human Rights Council (UNHRC), making it a report not endorsed by the international community.

It was issued again last year, but to no effect. Hence, one must ask, should there be any kind of diplomatic engagement between Pakistan and India? Because India has managed its Kashmir policy consistently, and it saddens me to say but, India has been moving methodically in order to make Pakistan irrelevant to the Kashmir dispute. India has also taken some measures within the occupied Jammu and Kashmir so the resistance is weakened from within.

We have seen over the last so many years as to how India has created forces to keep the resistance in check. It has also been successful in getting Hizbul Mujahideen – totally an indigenous resistance movement – proscribed by the US as a terrorist organization. So, even if talks begin tomorrow between Pakistan and India, I do not see India really budging from its position even an inch. I do not see diplomacy really working here and we are in a sad kind of situation.

I have been telling my own government that even if tomorrow, India reaches out to Pakistan, we should not engage with India at this point in time because such engagement would not result in anything, Unless and until there is some third-party mediation, to which India is unwilling.

President Donald Trump recently said that he is ready to mediate and so has the UN secretary general but India has refused and it has been refusing such ideas in the past. Thereby, there is no possibility of third-party mediation.

Bilateral engagement talks bear no fruit with India, too. The last bilateral dialogue framework was agreed between the two countries on December 9, 2015 in Islamabad, under the rubric of *Comprehensive Bilateral Dialogue* and under that rubric, India has taken a position; even objected to Pakistan's engagement with the Kashmiri leadership.

When I invited the Kashmiri leadership to the Pakistan High Commission in New Delhi, in August 2014, India objected. Subsequently, India's foreign secretary's visit to Pakistan was cancelled on that count. Similarly, our national security adviser was to visit India for meeting with his counterpart in August 2016.

Since our adviser wanted to meet the Hurriyat Conference leadership, the Indian government denied our national security adviser to visit India. So, over the years, especially under this government, this dispensation in India, India's position has hardened on Jammu and Kashmir.

They took this hard line from the Indian parliament's resolution of February 22, 1993, which not only talks about the occupied Jammu and Kashmir as an integral part, but also, talks about taking Azad Jammu and Kashmir, even if they have to use force.

We have seen that we couldn't have any UNSC meeting on Jammu and Kashmir after August 5, 2019, though we did have informal consultations. But that was not a formal meeting of the UNSC, which should have been open to both India and Pakistan.

We have also seen that even the Organization of Islamic Cooperation (OIC) has not been able to hold any special session on Jammu and Kashmir, though its contact group on Kashmir did meet several times, but there was no special session on Jammu and Kashmir as such as we have seen, they usually hold on Palestine and other issues.

Similarly, in the UNHRC, we could not even get 16 votes to have some discussion on Indian-occupied Kashmir. Thus, there is no international pressure on India and that is the biggest worry.

Thereby, unless there is international pressure on India, India is not going to give inalienable rights as was said to the people of Jammu and Kashmir in India. India usually accuses Pakistan of not abiding by its obligations under the UNSC resolutions and refers to a resolution that was passed by the United Nations Commission for India and Pakistan on August 13, 1948, that Pakistan would withdraw all its troops in order to facilitate the Kashmiris.

We always doubted the Indian intention and subsequently the UNSC adopted Resolution 98 on December 23, which allowed both, Pakistan and India, to retain their troops on both sides of Kashmir.

Legally and diplomatically speaking, Pakistan is on terra firma when it comes to Jammu and Kashmir but unfortunately, because of our inconsistencies; let me confess, we ourselves have weakened our position.

Originally, the MC Naughton Plan, Dickson Plan, and Chenab formula; they all came but we forgot about them. However, in 2004, when President Pervez Musharraf came up with his idea of four-point formula, it weakened our stance on Jammu and Kashmir, and disheartened the Kashmiris as well, especially those who were resisting Indian occupation.

Having lived and worked in India for almost four years, I have come to this conclusion that the entire KashmirsStruggle needs to be reorganized. And I highly doubt that political struggle alone would yield much for Kashmiris. It has to be juxtaposed with some kind of military resistance as pointed out by Dr. Shah. Let me add that there is an international principle, known as *erga omnes,* which binds the international community to help such struggles, and even provide military assistance, such as weapons, to such struggles, as was done by Pakistan.

As far international as law is concerned, armed struggle is legitimate. And Kashmiris cannot be denied of their right. Obviously, all of us want this problem to be resolved peacefully and nobody wants violence, but India has left Kashmiris and Pakistan with no other choice.

India continues procrastinating on Jammu and Kashmir; doesn't come to the negotiating table; doesn't realise that; and keeps on killing the people. Kashmiris have a strong case but, unfortunately, as I said earlier, I do not see any space for diplomacy really to work under the present circumstances.

Now, that the Indians have taken the biggest step they could – divided the state into two union territories against their own Constitution – what is left to talk about the UN Security Council resolutions? So, the situation has become more complex in my view, because in India, even if the BJP is not in power tomorrow, it would be very difficult for any other government.

The BJP will continue to be in power for some more time to come, and even if it is not in power, it will be very difficult for any other government to undo this step. Now that you know what has already been done by India, without resistance within occupied Kashmir dovetailed with the armed struggle, India will not come to the negotiating table to resolve this issue.

Session III

Classification of Atrocity Crimes Committed by Occupying Army in Indian-Occupied Kashmir

Dr. Patricia Hobbs[9]

Given the several crimes that have been perpetrated in Indian-occupied Kashmir (IOK), one would think that India is potentially liable, not just for human rights violations, but also potentially, for an international crime. I shall go through each of the crimes, starting with 'genocide', which is probably the least likely to actually find any potential for liability, not only in the context of state responsibility, but also in the context of 'individual criminal responsibility'.

India is not party to Rome Statute; therefore, it does not recognize and is not within the jurisdiction of the International Criminal Court. Of course, there's always a potential for the UNSC to send that situation to the ICC but that's very unlikely as well, given a potential veto by certain countries.

So, just to go through the actual crimes, I would start with genocide. And the reason I start with genocide is because it is certainly interesting from the viewpoint of the definition of genocide. It is exactly what is happening in IOK and to the population of IOK. Kashmiris are part recognized as indigenous people, and therefore, within the protection of the United Nations of *indigenous people* and according to this particular treaty, of course, the idea is: before anything is done within the territory of these people, there should be a free, prior, and informed consent to ensure that Kashmiris are actually exercising their sovereign indigenous rights as indigenous people. And of course, according to this

[9] Patricia Hobbs is lecturer in law, Brunel University. Her doctoral thesis focused on the relationship between Rome statute and the principle of state sovereignty. She has been regular judge in mooting competitions organized by Brunel University.

principle, all peoples have the right to self-determination, and obviously, linked to this right is the right to pursue economic, social and cultural development.

I've tied up genocide with this particular principle that applies specifically to indigenous people because the genocide convention, or rather the legal definition of genocide, is actually quite narrow; partly because, it does not provide an actual definition. It does not include cultural within its definition, although it does include ethnical. But ethnical, as we know, is not in itself very clear in the way that it is applied now. Also, if you go through the Article 6 of the Rome Statute, which reproduces verbatim the Article 2 of the Genocide Convention, there are certainly some of the elements there that could potentially be applied in the situation of IOK.

Detention, forcible transfer of people from Indian territory into the IOK territory, arbitrary imprisonment of individuals, inhumane and degraded treatment, and severe torture are dire crimes being committed by the Indian state. But, the problem is: the definition is narrow and it does not allow for potentially what is happening in IOK. Potentially it could fit within one of those acts of the genocide as a genocide convention of the Rome's older statute.

But as you know, in practice, genocide is hard to prove. And one of the problems with genocide is the intent. So, unless you have that special intent to commit that particular crime, which is of course, the intent to destroy the whole part of a national ethnical, racial, or religious group; it is quite difficult to actually find a liability under Genocide Convention.

In recent years, actually after the 1990s, there have been findings of genocide in the context of Rwanda and in the context of the former Yugoslavia. For example, it was only in the context of Sherbin that a finding of genocide was actually upheld by the International Court of Justice. This was about state responsibility as opposed to individual responsibility, but we need other cases that go ahead with regard to genocide from the viewpoint of individual criminal responsibility. We need that in the context of Bosnia versus Serbia and also Croatia versus Serbia. Although some of the acts committed did amount to the Soviet race of genocide itself, but there was not enough evidence to actually find that there was a special intent to destroy in whole or in part a certain group of people.

The International Criminal Tribunal for the former Yugoslavia (ICTY), again in the context of the former Yugoslavia, did find a number of cases related and did uphold in the context of genocide, abetting genocide. So, in the context of IOK, it would probably be the least likely to prove genocide, successfully. It is partly because of the 'special intent' and the way the legal definition is constructed now.

The situation in IOK is similar to what's going on in Israel and Palestine. And the way Israel has quietly occupied the Palestinian territory and perpetrated a number of human rights violations in that territory. There are, of course, suggestions for some writers that this is a slow move to genocide; it's not as quick and as clear as it was happening in Rwanda; or as it happened in the context of the former Yugoslavia. It's more insidious than that. As I study more about the academic, theoretical discussion, I wonder if, in fact, there could be any liability on India for genocide and for the acts perpetrated by India in the IOK territory.

There are other discussions that are quite interesting here with regard to genocide, including the original viewpoint or the original vision by Raphael Lemkin. When he came up with the label of genocide, it did not go far with the final definition, and did not cover certain groups of people that he originally intended to include.

Now, 'crimes against humanity' is certainly different because crimes against humanity offer the possibilities of the fact that they can be committed both, in times of war and in times of peace. So, you don't have the extra burden of having to prove whether there is an armed conflict or not. More so, you do not need to debate whether the conflict is international or non-international, which, in itself, leads to other problems and issues. Seeking attention for the crimes against humanity has got thus, an extra advantage.

Anyway, whether India ratifies the Rome Statute or not, it would be bound to some extent, to answer and be held accountable for behavior and the acts it commits against the people of IOK. So, when you're talking about torture, rape, sexual crimes, murder, enslavement, and persecution, it would certainly attract some element of attention, because, persecution is identified as a group or collectivity on political, racial, national, ethnic, cultural, religious, and gender as defined in paragraph three of the Rome Statute.

However, the elements here that need to be satisfied are the contextual elements. First of all, we have this sort of a notion of 'attack' that may be difficult to actually define in practice and whether the court's definition of *attack* would actually match what the Indian forces are doing on the ground in IOK. To incite any legal attention, this attack needs to be part of a widespread and systematic action, directed against any civilian population. So, the idea that it needs to be widespread and systematic does not elaborate if 'widespread' is limited to the concept of numbers. 'Widespread' could also refer to territory itself. It is, in part, sort of a wider government agenda in furtherance of some sort of policy to commit such attack.

In some ways, some of the elements here are potentially fulfilled. The 'attack' in itself may be questioned. What India has done, I'm sure India would defend it in the context of sovereignty. India has taken the action to implement particular laws and to effectively annex IOK into Indian Territory. From this point of view, if you look at some of the cases, especially, post Rwanda and Yugoslavia, with the International Criminal Tribunal for Rwanda (ICTR) and ICTY, there are some very vivid examples of crimes against humanity. The one that I would specifically point out is what happened in Kenya. In terms of magnitude, it may not be an apt comparison, because I'm not quite sure about the actual civil unrest in Kenya at that time. But I am aware of the actions taken by India against IOK.

There was civil unrest in Kenya after an election, and that in itself was deemed to be a crime against humanity. And effectively, in that particular episode, it was found to be systematic. About a thousand people were actually killed in that unrest. In the context of the civil unrest in Kenya, potentially, the world may *actually* find crimes against humanity in IOK, being committed by India.

As I mentioned before, one of the problems with the finding of war crime is: there needs to be basis for acknowledgement an international armed conflict. It seems to me that India has got an interesting and maybe more traditional perspective on state sovereignty. I've noticed that it has entered some declarations albeit resembling reservations with regard to the International Covenant on Civil and Political Rights (ICCPR) and the International Covenant on Economic, Social and Cultural Rights (ICESCR) and it's not party to the Geneva Convention, Additional Protocols of 1977. So, from that point of view, we can quickly establish that India would try very hard to contest that there was no international armed conflict. Even if the IOK issue is portrayed as a domestic non-international armed conflict, it is still perpetrated by India, and could still amount to violation of Common Article 3.

Lastly, 'crime of aggression' is very interesting. I'll go back to the ICC, which obviously can have jurisdiction for this particular crime, which also includes occupation.

India, of course, was clever in a way to adjust the Constitution and amend some of its domestic laws. But, for all intents and purposes, this is an annexation of IOK into India. And with the amount of forces that India actually sent to IOK, it can only amount to an occupation, which would be covered by the crime of aggression, listed in *Article* 8 of the Rome Statute. And, of course, if it is an occupation, India has to comply with the Geneva Convention, the fourth conventional convention with regard to the protection afforded.

Having said that, Geneva Convention 4 is applicable, just like all conventions, on international armed conflicts, apart from the minimal amount of human rights protection, offered by Article 3 itself.

In conclusion, it's not just clear-cut; it's insidious; and it's similar, as I said, to what's happening between Israel and Palestinian. The issue is: self-defense against terrorism etc. very similar to some of the propositions put forward by the Indian government.

Thus, the route to the ICC would actually be quite hard unless you have a referral by the Security Council. So, the other avenue would have to be a different court, a domestic court, which would decide to exercise jurisdiction on the universal jurisdiction. Again, that would be quite difficult, but not impossible. Thereby, as I have said before, 'crimes against humanity' may indeed be the best way forward. And that concludes my discussion.

Threshold of Armed Conflict in IOK

Prof. Abdul Rauf Khatana[10]

Does this conflict fall within the jargon of International Humanitarian Law (IHL)? Is it an international armed conflict or not? Let us analyze whether the ongoing situation in IOK meets the threshold of International Armed Conflict or not.

Let us see if war crimes or alleged genocide, and some of the other violations are systematic and the gross violations of the international human rights as well. Once these crimes are established, as Dr. Patricia Hobbs mentioned, they will attract some of the provisions. Indeed, India *is* committing these crimes. This is not only a Pakistani stance or Kashmiri view, independent observers from the UN, and other independent agencies, have also substantiated this disposition.

But, how to deal with these crimes since these crimes are heinous? If war crimes are being committed; if genocide is being committed; if systematic violation of human rights is going on; and being prolonged; how can it be dealt with? And

the answer to this question is in the international law, particularly and particularly, in the International Humanitarian Law.

Yes, we can find answers to this question in international law, International Human Rights Law, and IHL, as well. But let us focus on the IHL for the moment.

I believe that this is an international armed conflict. One may wonder: why should we call it an international armed conflict, and what if we do not call this an international armed

[10] Abdur Rauf Khattana is Assistant Professor of Law, LL.M in Human Rights, Conflict and Justice (SOAS, UK), MA in Philosophy (University of Peshawar).

conflict? The atrocities are the violations of the human rights as mentioned earlier, which are ceaseless in the valley. There are two parties in this conflict: one is a state with force, while the other are people, the weaker party. Law is supposed to protect the weaker party and in this regard, we being academics, believe that it is our academic responsibility to point out the most appropriate and accurate law, which can deal with the situation.

I will try to categorize my points from the perspective of the weaker party, as well as, from the perspective of the state – the powerful party. Geneva Conventions use the term *high contracting powers* for such parties. The stronger party, or the state, or the aggressor, will always brand such situations as a kind of domestic and internal disturbance. And they would always propose that their domestic law is capable to deal with the situation. They deny some of the violations of the human rights or some of the other civil liberties. And they always come up with the same rebuttal: there's a Constitution and domestic law, which can address and provide remedies to the aggrieved party.

All is well from India's perspective. But the fact of the matter is: we will not call it just domestic or internal disturbance. The activities which are going on there, the situation from the perspective of the weaker party, from the perspective of those who are victims, and who are at the receiving end, it is far from just an internal disturbance. Obviously, India will not accept it as an international armed conflict. The scope of the law or the scope of the regulations, which can address the issue from the perspective of weaker party is the application of Common Article 3 that provides certain remedies for the situations which do not fall within the international armed conflict criterion. They are categorized as non-international. Even then, though if this is recognized, the weaker party, and the liberation movement will get some sort of remedies for them.

But if we successfully establish that it is, indeed, an international armed conflict, the whole of IHL comes to be enforced, and it will certainly take care of the weaker party because the weaker party is in disregard. That is why the stronger party is denying this position. Any party occupying a particular territory will obviously not accept that this is an international armed conflict, because the whole range of IHL, including the Geneva Conventions, and Additional Protocols, and Customary International Law will come up to point out their inhuman acts – the war crimes and the violations of the human rights committed by them.

This is precisely why India denies the status of this conflict as an international armed conflict.

When I take this position that this is the international armed conflict, I am precisely relying on two agents, and these two agents are obviously from the IHL and the Geneva Conventions. The very first article, which I would like to quote, is *Article 2*. It is common to all the four Geneva Conventions. Article 2 says, *"In addition to the provisions which have been implemented in peacetime, the present convention shall apply."* It is common to all the conventions. It refers that all the four conventions shall apply to all cases of declared war, or any other armed conflict, which may arise between two or more of high contracting parties. I would like to go beyond this; it continues and says, *"even if the state of war is not recognized by one of them, and then the second paragraph the Convention shall also apply to all cases of partial or total occupation of the territory of a high contracting party, even if the said occupation meets with no armed resistance."*

I would drag your attention to the occupation. The word *occupation* has been used here, in cases of occupation where one high contracting party is occupying. Hence, armed conflict in IOK meets the threshold of an international armed conflict, and it covers the application of all the four Geneva Conventions, because this is particularly common to all the four conventions.

One may ask that on what basis can India be qualified as an occupying force here? Let us substantiate this proposition. First of all, when the partition took place in 1947, the principle, precisely, was that the princely states shall decide on their own, whether they want to accede with Pakistan or India. Kashmir was admittedly a princely state, and there is no denial of the effect from either of the parties to the conflict.

India pleads that the Maharaja submitted or rendered the deed of accession and, by virtue of that, IOK became an integral part of India. On the other hand, the other position is that the deed of accession was not recognized *legal* in the light of international law. There are many things which have been mentioned and much has been written on this by many people. I would like to refer to Dr. Ijaz Hussain's book, *Kashmir dispute: An international law perspective.*

According to him, the deal of accession is not legally valid in the eyes of international law, and alleged that it was signed under duress. The Maharaja did not even exercise it in accordance with the wishes of the people. It is a well-known fact that the majority of the population was Muslim, and the Muslims of Kashmir wanted to accede with Pakistan.

When this issue was taken to the UN because of a conflict which took place in 1948 between India and Pakistan, in one of its earlier resolutions, the United Nations Security Council provided that the issue shall be resolved in accordance with the wishes of the people through a referendum. This was accepted by both India and Pakistan. At that point, India did not assert the position that there was a deed of accession. And, according to the agreement upon the princely states, these states were on their own to decide whether they would join India or Pakistan.

The UN Charter does not provide any criterion for the right of self-determination directly. But some points and some criteria have been mentioned in the covenants. If you go through *Article 1*, you will see *"All peoples have the right of self-determination. By virtue of that right they freely determine their political status and freely pursue their economic, social and cultural development. All peoples may, for their own ends, freely dispose of their natural wealth and resources without prejudice to any obligations arising out of international economic co-operation, based upon the principle of mutual benefit, and international law. In no case may a people be deprived of its own means of subsistence."*

Hence, the IHRL, for the reference of definition, mentions that whenever and wherever there is economic exploitation, exploitation of the civil liberties, exploitation of the fundamental rights; the people of that community have the right of self-determination. Without going into the rhetoric of what is *the right of self-determination,* I would like to mention, the UNSC, in its resolutions, has had admitted this right of self-determination for the people of Kashmir in *Resolution 47* of April 21, 1948, where especially the right of self-determination for the people of Kashmir was mentioned and recognized. And, it was reiterated in the subsequent resolutions from the UNSC. Once the right of self-determination is recognized, keeping in view the provision of *Additional Protocol 1, Sub-Article 4,* it meets the threshold of the International Armed Conflict.

Thereby, the persisting situation *does* fall within the very definition of *international armed conflict.*

Azad Jammu and Kashmir Post-August 5, 2019

Farzana Yaqoob[11]

We must admit that we are very late in this game, but at least, the young Kashmiris have taken this responsibility upon themselves of not depending on others to speak about them. They are looking for solutions themselves.

The most important part for me is not just that we might be able to find some kind of legal solution or otherwise, but the fact that it is you who's providing the vocabulary to the discussion on Kashmir.

Be it war crimes or occupying force, these words were seldom used. But now, because of organizations such as the LFK, it is becoming a common understanding that the issue of Kashmir is an International Armed Conflict.

The LFK is a success, and we must have these sessions as regularly as possible, because our understanding improves when we have such intellectual debates where speakers try not only explaining these issues but also provide a solution, and share a way forward.

Let us look at the situation in Azad Jammu and Kashmir after India abrogated the special status of Indian-occupied Kashmir on August 5, 2019.

Whenever a human rights report is issued, for example two recent reports by the UNHRC, it not only highlights the issues in Indian-occupied Kashmir but also contains a few reservations on Azad Jammu and Kashmir based on the assumption that media here is not completely free.

---

[11] Farzana Yaqoob is the Founding Member of the Asia Institute of Public Policy and is a Policy Advisor for AGAHI. She formerly served as Minister for Social Welfare and Women Development in Azad Jammu and Kashmir, having been elected in 2011. She is also an Eisenhower Fellow (2016); her focus during the fellowship was on conflict resolution and climate change mitigation strategies.

During the last one year at least, any foreigner visiting Azad Jammu and Kashmir would require a No Objection Certificate (NOC) from Pakistan's Ministry of Interior.

Though Azad Kashmir is a peaceful place, when you require an NOC, it means that there could be a security situation. This implies that the threat level in Azad Jammu and Kashmir is always high, mainly because of the cross-border firing along the Line of Control (LoC), a de facto border between India and Pakistan that divides the Himalayan valley.

We must address the issues that are highlighted by the UNHCR in its 2020 report. The issue of NOC, at least to my understanding, was removed. I was making arrangements for a foreign journalist to visit Azad Kashmir in 2019, and on the last day we found out that an NOC was no longer required.

Another issue is the State Subject Certificate, which identifies a Kashmiri. But, for an international identification, the people of Azad Kashmir have Pakistani passports, while those in IOK carry Indian passports. This is why when our Kashmiri brothers and sisters have to enter Pakistan, they face problems. And this is something we need to resolve not only at Azad Jammu and Kashmir level, but also at the legislative level in Pakistan.

The LoC, even during the best of times, is a dangerous place. Civilians on both sides of the border are caught in the crossfire. They have families.

For us, family means brothers and sisters, nephews and nieces, extended families, as well as close friends. The bloodline of the tribe is a family. So, maybe a sister's family is on this side and her brother's on the other.

When armies fight, it is the civilians that suffer the most.

One is often asked, why do people live in conflict zones? It is difficult for people to leave their ancestral lands. People prefer their native land. Kashmiris would die defending it.

India is trying to usurp our territory, as well as trying to erase our identity.

It does not even respect the white flag for ambulances to pass through. It is difficult for internatonal observers to visit. Any such trip to be organized requires security protocols since Indian forces can start shelling any time.

One thing positive was the establishment of a joint chamber of commerce, and joint association of journalists and lawyers. But all went in vain after August 5.

We must find some way where any local, national, or international association or organization could help the Kashmiris. We need to come up with some kind of instrument, which does not block Kashmiris from meeting in person.

The situation in Kashmir has gone from bad to worse over the decades. Even before 1947, the state was violated by colonial masters and their loyal servants. Kashmiris are continuously suffering.

Yet, Kashmiris have never accepted occupation.

I hope we come up with some kind of solution. Till the Kashmiris are alive, this issue will remain alive. Kashmiris will not let it die until and unless it is resolved.

I wanted to keep it as short as possible, and just wanted to share what is happening at the local level, and how the situation can be improved.

Session IV

Status of Indigenous Armed Groups Fighting for Right to Self-Determination

Prof. Sikander Ahmed Shah[12]

In the context of IOK, there are two things that demand delineation: self-determination, and the status of the movement of freedom fighters, under the law of armed conflicts.

Let us look at the law of self-determination. In a way, it is outside the ambit of IHL law. The right to self-determination and the armed struggle for freedom are intertwined and related to each other. Because, in order to realize the right of self-determination in IOK, the only viable option for the people of IOK is to move on, not just in peaceful ways but also through armed struggle. And for that, it is important to understand the legal paradigm of the armed struggle, which would discuss the law of armed conflict. We need to characterize and understand the ways and methods in which the Kashmiris are fighting the Indian occupation.

Self-determination is a recognized right under the international law, and has increasingly become a part of the international customary norm. The reason why it is, still in some sense, subservient or undermined is: the right of sovereignty, which is the primordial or the most important norm of international law. The international system is solely based on it. Once the state realizes its independence, the law of sovereignty is applicable for it. But a lot of nations and states, and a lot of people are under occupation. So, the law of sovereignty is often misused, as India does, to undermine the cause of the Kashmiri freedom struggle.

[12] Professor Sikander Shah is a pioneering member of the Shaikh Ahmad Hassan School of Law, LUMS. Professor Shah served as the Legal Advisor to the Ministry of Foreign Affairs, while he was on sabbatical in 2012-2013. Professor Shah's teaching and research interests are focused on Public International Law, International Human Rights Law, International Humanitarian Law, Corporate Governance and Constitutional Design.

Freedom struggle is the right that is recognized not just under the Customary Law, but also in various UN General Assembly resolutions, as well as UNSC resolutions under *Chapter VI*. Subsequently, as recognized by the majority of the world community, there's no doubt that Kashmiris have a right to self-determination.

The UN Charter, which now reflects the Customary International Law in all its forms, mentions the right to self-determination under Article 1. It is the first article that recognizes the right to self-determination of people. However, it does not define it. The definition comes under the Common Article 1 of both, the UN and the ICESCR. Both of these are now read under the Customary International Law. And these conventions, in detail, give people an inalienable right to define and determine their political status, and freely pursue their economic, social, and cultural development. They have the right to use their own natural resources, which in the case of IOK, as we know, has *not* happened. India is exploiting IOK's resources, and political rights, both from a self-determined and also from an internal self-determination perspective.

All people living under the control of a particular country or a state must have access to basic universal human rights. If those rights are undermined, the right of internal self-determination eventually graduates to the right of external self-determination.

The right to self-determination is also discussed under *Article 55* of the UN Charter, which is about the promotion of rights such as standard of living, employment, economic and social progress, development, cultural rights, education, respect for human rights, and no distinction based on race, sex, language, or religion. Even in this context, the right to self-determination is recognized.

Moving forward, the right is recognized under Customary Law as well, which is also reflected through UN General Assembly Resolutions on self-determination, the most prominent being *UNGA Res 2625* – the declaration on principle of international friendly relations and cooperation among states. It clearly lists and recognizes the right to self-determination. In this context, the right to an armed struggle is also recognized. *Resolutions 122, 2625, 2649* and other prominent UNGA resolutions discuss this right.

The writers also discussed ICJ judgments including advisory opinion on Libya, West Africa. The cases concerning the frontier dispute of Burkina Faso, Republic of Mali, and Eastern Portugal versus Australia are worth mentioning here. Portugal versus Australia is rather a recent judgment. It establishes: one of the essential principles of Customary International Law is being recognized as the customary norm.

So the right to self-determination, as applicable on IOK is recognized under UNSC resolutions because India itself is the country that took this matter to the UN. Subsequently, there is a particular chapter in the resolution that deals with specific settlements of the dispute, which never happened.

Before I discuss the law of armed conflict with regards to self-determination, I must state that the right to self-determination has been further undermined by Indian authorities now, through the revocation of certain constitutional provisions.

The arrangements with people and Kashmiri leaders, who were pro-India, are now being reneged. We are moving further away from what India had been claiming, or has claimed, and what they had agreed to. India is also walking away from the declaration which talks about not changing the status quo in any way.

Moving to the armed conflict and the role of freedom fighters in IOK, one must not ignore that they avail protections. An occupation is defined under Common *Article 2* of the Geneva Conventions. One can see a more detailed definition in the *Article 42 of the Hague Convention of 1907*. I quote, *"Territory is considered occupied when it is actually placed under the authority of the hostile army. The occupation extends only to the territory where such authority has been established and can be exercised."* The *Fourth Geneva*

Convention indicts India of occupation in Kashmir. While India hasn't ratified or signed the Fourth Geneva Convention, the Convention is now considered Customary International Law. India is in violation of observation law also, in terms of crimes discussed so forth. These are war crimes that India is systematically and historically committing in occupied territories.

India argues that Kashmiris are not combatants in the real sense because you have combatants only in international armed conflicts. Clearly, this is an incorrect interpretation of the situation. First of all, Indian-occupied Kashmir (IOK) is not a territory of India. It was always a princely state and always had its right to join either India or Pakistan, or remain independent, as established by the UNSC.

This is not a situation where you have what would be a purely non-international armed conflict, where there is some discretion on states to not define combatants as combatants, but as organized armed groups. It shouldn't make any difference because *Additional Protocol 1 (AP-1)* and *Additional Protocol 2 (AP-2)* are applicable to non-national armed conflicts. AP-1 applies to international armed conflict and a lot of the definitions coming from AP-1 are now considered Customary International Law, even though, India and Pakistan have not signed AP-1 or AP-2. In terms of domestic law also, there are various understandings of what combatants are. Why is it important to define combatants? Combatants have privileges, and are considered civilians.

If you look at the UNGA, it doesn't really make these distinctions in the 1970 General Assembly resolution. It speaks of combatants in all armed conflicts. A combatant is defined by organization, complying with the laws of war which the IHL expressed. Kashmiris are merely fighters. When they target Indian forces, they target proportionally. They don't use unnecessary force and they don't target civilians, like the India forces do. They also do not use any banned weapons, which the Indian army uses, such as pellet guns. They distinguish between combatants and civilians by targeting Indian armed forces, whereas, there are numerous cases of India targeting civilians on a regular basis. So, there is no reason to take away the status of Kashmiri fighters as not being combatants.

In terms of calling Kashmiri fighters as combatants, or using language of the IHL of belligerent occupation, the right to self-defense or the right of using force to realize the right to self-defense is completely legal. Using the IHL language and the narrative of IHL, Kashmiri fighters or combatants comply with laws of war; their use of force (A 2(4) UN Charter) is proportionally necessary. They do not use banned weapons and they do not cause unnecessary suffering. They use force for when it is a military necessity, which is defined under the Geneva Conventions and the Additional Protocols for the Geneva Conventions.

Henceforth, an armed force with the objective of gaining a definite military advantage is doing nothing illegal if it fights for the realization of the right of self-determination.

Kashmir Conflict and Applicable International Humanitarian Laws

Sami-ur-Rehman[13]

It was discussed that this conflict has the nature of occupation and the law of occupation is applicable to the ongoing conflict in IOK.

But I have something different in my mind to ease the difficulties of Kashmiri people, who have been suffering at the hands of Indian occupying forces since 1948. If we call it an occupation, it becomes an issue of International Armed Conflict. Thereby, all the

[13] Sami ur Rehman is assistant professor at shariah academy.

Geneva Conventions, additional protocols, Customary International Law, and International Criminal Law will become applicable to the situation of occupation.

For me, to ease the difficulties of the Kashmiri people, and to give them the bare minimum safeguards and safeties available under the IHL, under the armed conflict would be the classification of this conflict as non-international armed conflict. The IHL is applicable to all conflict situations, whether the conflict is of international character or not, but the legal regime for these two types of conflicts, is different because to be qualified as an international armed conflict, the conflict has to be between two or more than two states.

All the four Geneva Conventions, Additional Protocol 1, Hague Law and International Criminal Law are all applicable to international armed conflicts, and together, they govern the modalities of warfare, war crimes, and their consequences. Convincing India of the application of these bulky laws is next to impossible. But, what we can do is to convince the Indian government, to at least give the Kashmiris the fundamental guarantees being provided in Common Article 3 to the four Geneva Conventions, additional protocol, and the Customary IHL.

Common Article 3 is quite common, and it is known as the mini convention, because it provides so many guarantees to the people who are fighting within a state territory. In non-international conflicts, for example, there are four bare minimum guarantees available to everyone. Violence to life and person, in particular, murder of all kinds, mutilation, cruel treatment, and torture are prohibited under *Common Article 3*. India is violating the life of people, killing them, murdering them, mutilating them. The freedom fighters are routinely arrested, cruelly treated, and inhumanely tortured. Torture is an issue of human rights law and humanitarian law, equally. One cannot deny this prohibition to anyone. Thus, if we are simply saying that the conflict of IOK should be considered as a non-international armed conflict, then the Indian forces and the Indian government is responsible to prohibit its soldiers from committing violence to life.

Second guarantee, available in *Common Article 3* is about hostages. Indian army cannot take any person as a hostage for any purposes.

The third guarantee is an outrage upon personal dignity, in particular, humiliating and degrading treatment. Degrading or humiliating is declared as prohibited in *Common Article 3.*

Fourth is related to some judicial guarantees. It is one of the fundamental guarantees available under *Common Article 3* of the four Geneva Conventions. It says that the passing of sentences and carrying out of executions, without prior announcement of the judgment by a regularly constituted court, affording all the judicial guarantees, which are recognized as indispensable by civilized people, is prohibited.

I'm not talking about AP-2 because India has not signed or ratified it. The AP- 2 has been called *"the Bible of terrorists"*. The US administration gave it the title since there are so many guarantees available to the belligerents, insurgents who are fighting against their governments, within the territory of one state.

Since, India has not signed it, the international community cannot insist to implement whatever has been guaranteed in additional protocols. This is a legal hurdle for us. But there is another way out for the application of these fundamental guarantees, and that way out is the application of Customary IHL. Customary IHL is applicable to each and every situation, whether it is an international conflict or not. In each and every situation, the rules of Customary IHL have to be implemented. The Indian government, and its forces are obliged to follow the fundamental rules of the Customary International Law.

Combatants who surrender and civilians, both are to be treated humanely. This is the *Rule 90 of the Customary IHL. Rule 93* says that torture and cruel, inhuman treatment, and outrage upon personal dignity, in particular, humanity, are prohibited. In *Common Article 3*, rape and other forms of sexual violence are prohibited. Rape is one kind of battle a method of means of warfare, which should be, of course, immediately stopped. There are thousands of incidents of rape in IOK, which is of course prohibited and this is the violation of the Customary IHL.

Enforced disappearance is also prohibited. This is mentioned in *Rule 98* of the Customary IHL. We all know that Kashmiris in IOK are suffering from this type of disappearances on a daily basis. This should halt at once. In the fifth guarantee, which is available to each and every one under Customary International Law – Arbitrary Deprivation of Liberty – prohibits this, too.

Sixth is that no one may be convicted or sentenced except pursuant to fair trial affording all necessary judicial guarantees, and we know that no such fair judicial guarantees are available to anyone living and residing in the IOK.

Seventh guarantee suggests that the convictions and religious practices of civilians and combatants must be respected.

Eighth fundamental guarantee, available in the Customary IHL, claims that mutilation, medical or scientific experiments, or any other procedure not indicated by the state of health of the person concerned, and not consistent with the generally accepted medical standards are prohibited. But the people that are being taken are being experimented upon. They are being exposed to some medical and scientific experiments which are not in accordance with the humanity.

Ninth guarantee states that uncompensated abuse and abusive or forced labor are prohibited. The detaining power cannot ask you for such forced labor or which is uncompensated for. So, if you are involved in labor, you have to be compensated, which is also guaranteed by Customary Law in relation to the armed conflict.

Hostage taking is also prohibited, which is the repetition of what we just mentioned in Common Article 3 and Article 75 of the AP-1 of course. The AP-1 again is not signed by India. In any case, the fundamental guarantees identified in Article 75 are the repetition of Rule 90. There are also some rules related to the protection of people who are not fighting, who are the civilian population. Thereby, if someone has been taken away by the forces, he or she must be given proper means of defense. So he or she should be able to defend him or herself. A person can be convicted only on the basis of individual criminal responsibility.

The last interpretation of what is mentioned in the rules of CIHL and the *Common Article 3* is: accused is innocent, until proved guilty. *Article 4 of the Hague Regulation* describes the features of a combatant. There are four features, if someone fulfils, he or she could be considered as a combatant. But, there is a huge technical issue related to the status of a combatant in international conflicts and non-international conflicts. However, the baseline remains the same. The baseline of this law is humanity. Humanity must prevail in each and every crisis.

Therefore, the application of the combatant status in international armed conflict confers upon you the right to be considered as a prisoner of war (POW), which is of course, is a prestigious status, and has been protected under *the Geneva Convention 3 of 1949*. But, if you are fighting, and you are an insurgent, and a belligerent, you are not entitled to the status of POWs, if caught, because the *Geneva Convention 3* is only applicable in case of international conflicts.

There are four criteria set out in Hague Regulations which qualify you as a combatant: that you carry arms openly, you are under a responsible command, you carry and wear a weapon which makes you distinguished from the civilians, and you obey the rules and regulations of the law of warfare. While fighting with the Indian forces the Kashmiris have never used banned weapons; they have never detained any civilian population. They have never committed atrocities against the opponent army: neither took Indian armed forces personnel to prison camps nor tortured them. I have never come across any such reports or findings.

What we need to do in the contemporary situation is to pursue our case in such a way that India gives Kashmiris the bare minimum fundamental. And that's how we would move towards getting more benefits, from the current legal regime, applicable to the conflict situation in IOK.

Indian Military Occupation of Kashmir and Available Legal Remedies

Raja Sajjad Khan[14]

During the last few years, we have changed our narrative constantly. We have been changing our legal phrases and terminologies. This has changed the context of the conflict in Indian-occupied Kashmir. We should understand that in legal warfare, the prime objective of our efforts should be the internationalization of this case in its true legal context.

We should keep in mind the legal implications and the legal output of our effort, and when we say that the situation in IOK is an international armed conflict, there are two dimensions to this conflict. First: it is a conflict between India and Pakistan; the armies of both the countries are under a cease-fire, which is frequently violated and results in civilian casualties. Hence, it is not only an international armed conflict, but also a threat to peace and stability.

At the same time the struggle is indigenous, and the pro-freedom leadership is fighting to achieve their right to self-determination.

---

[14] Raja Sajjad Khan is director Jammu Kashmir Liberation cell, Government of Azad Jammu Kashmir and PHD scholar IIUI.

Multiple reports by international human rights organizations have revealed that India is committing crimes against humanity, and breaching the IHL under the Customary International Law in the occupied valley, as discussed previously; and the Four Geneva Conventions and the additional protocols.

Both Islamabad and Muzaffarabad need to develop a joint strategy against military occupation of IOK. For this purpose, Pakistan should provide political, diplomatic, and logistic support to Kashmiris on the other side of the border.

Secondly, the aspect of their right to self-determination should continue to be pursued. Thirdly, after August 5, 2019, the role of Azad Jammu and Kashmir has become more important because it is the only government representing the people of Jammu and Kashmir.

The government of the union territory, nominated and installed by the Indian government, does not represent Kashmiris. Muzaffarabad should lead the campaign and Pakistan should provide all the assistance in this regard. Pakistan should also exercise its legal options within the context of international conventions.

When we discuss if the case should be built on the basis of human rights violations or genocide, the basic problem we face is Pakistan's approval of the applicable conventions. We should analyze and discuss the political and legal implications for ratification of different conventions and charters.

The Kashmiri diaspora should be supported to invoke the last universal jurisdiction. There are many cases of human rights violations in IOK that have been reported and well documented, and the victims' family members are living in the UK or Brussels. They can invoke the universal jurisdiction law there, and we should prepare a case on these grounds.

The next suggestion is that we are only focusing on the political forum; we should establish legal and academic forums as well, which can play an important part in projection of the Kashmir cause.

Legal experts and research scholars should analyze the model of Turkish Republic of Northern Cyprus and Morocco National Liberation Army. Both have observer status in the Organization of Islamic Cooperation (OIC) and we should analyze these two cases with the case of Azad Jammu and Kashmir government and look into how we can project these two governments in line with these two organizations, and see if it is in the interest of the people of IOK and Pakistan.

Pakistan should announce its withdrawal from the Simla Agreement, which has been violated after India's unilateral decision on August 5, 2019.

These are some of my suggestions. We all are convinced that Kashmir is an international armed conflict. We need to frame and establish this case on legal grounds internationally.

Role of United Nations to Address the Prolonged Indian Military Occupation of Kashmir

Catherine Constantinides[15]

As an activist, I came to Azad Jammu and Kashmir exactly a year ago. Coming from South Africa, a country with bleak history, it is important to note that we are a young democracy of only 25 years. Our perspective based on our new-found democratic norms allows us to feel nostalgic, seeing the situation in Indian-occupied Kashmir, and many lessons can be derived here.

We are seeing an occupation in IOK; we are seeing a lockdown, which is in place for over a year. The media blackout is real. The clampdown has resulted in the loss of so many lives, and we have seen people not being able to connect with their families, having no idea of the situation or the well-being of their loved ones.

Coming from South Africa, a country in Africa, where there are so many different kinds of conflicts, but only one colony – the colony of Western Sahara – under the military occupation by Morocco. I must lay stress that the United Nations is not the only body that can serve us, and give us the answers that we are looking for. We have to fight, to continue keeping the issue of Kashmir, Western Sahara, Palestine, and many others on the agenda.

We need to ensure that conversations and debates such as these happening today must happen on a vast platform and on a continual basis. We need to make sure that awareness and education are a priority, and we must continue to educate and create awareness of what the issue of IOK is. We understand that the media is globally controlled by the elite, who are trying to ensure that the world only knows what they want them to know.

[15]Catherine is an international speaker. A Humanitarian, Human Rights Defender and Climate, environmental & Social Justice Activist.

Therefore, the IOK issue is not out and on global networks and platforms it is given minimal mainstream media coverage and publicity.

We need grass-root-level organizations, the academics, and social movements and bodies. Not only in Pakistan, but also in regions around the globe, we need to continue to talk about Kashmir.

Five years ago, I started to work at the United Nations Human Rights Council (UNHRC), specifically working on the illegal occupation and the fight for self-determination of the people of Western Sahara, and it was there that I first came into contact with Kashmiri activists and the conflict in IOK. What is going on behind the curtains – the violations of human rights via torture; very specifically, the mutilation; the torture; the rape of women and children – is something that horrified me. It horrified me because far down south on the other tip of Africa, in South Africa, where I come from, this is not an issue that is brought to the forefront. It is not something that we continually talk about or even care about. So, minimal information is known about this specific conflict.

Those who are reading this, I would really encourage you to not only share the information that you are taking away, but continue to share it in a way that you can educate your own communities, and social media.

Technology has allowed us communicate easily. I'm on the other end of the world and I'm able to be with you. As an activist, I can say that we need to fight through the United Nations. We must not only work as academics, we need to cross-reference all the work that we're doing, and we need to broaden the understanding of the issue of IOK, far across different specters of people, social communities, and organizations around the world. They need to start talking about the illegal occupations that still exists in the year 2020. Torture, murder, rape, and mutilation cannot continue to happen on our watch. We see ourselves as such a forward-moving human race and yet we are destroying the lives of the people every single day.

Names of people, who die, go unknown to the world. We must not tolerate that the global media's agenda is only what serves a few who have money and power. We cannot allow global powerhouses such as India to control the media. We need to put a stop to this and the only way we will do it is from the ground up, and therefore, I would encourage you to continue using your platforms.

Everyone has access to some kind of platform via Twitter, Facebook, Instagram etc. Continue sharing information. Let us dispel fake information and fake news that continues to fill and flood all of our timelines. We need all to be activists.

The use of correct maps is vitally important in our fight for Western Sahara and the self-determination of the Saharawi people. Maps are incredibly important. Every time we see an incorrect map, either up on a wall or printed somewhere, we need to take action. We need to ask for the removal of those incorrect maps. We need to make sure that we are putting out the correct information that the world needs to see. We need to be the ones that are telling the stories.

This is the longest protracted occupation in modern history. How can it be that this continues to happen? We can send a man to the moon, but we are unable to ensure the inalienable right of self-determination for the IOK people or for the Saharawi people or for the Palestinians; and the list goes on.

I would encourage you all to continue being activists from the corners that you live in. It is important that we keep constant communication. We need to ensure that we are communicating correct information. We are using the WhatsApp groups that are available to us to constantly share news that goes out, with broader spectra of people. Let us widen our circle; let us ensure that the next time we meet under this wonderful forum, and thanks to the organizers to organize such talks that are very important; let us do this again in some weeks' time. But let us make sure that we have expanded this specific platform as an activist who fights for human rights and social justice. It is important for me to see that more people know about the IOK conflict, and more people are aware.

When people see news, articles or paging through a newspaper, depending on where in the world you are, there should be a column that talks about specific issues on the ground and need to tell your stories. And as an activist, I would encourage that, because I can only learn from you to be able to do so much more to use the platforms.

I have to continue working and fighting and bringing life to the specific issue. They are the legal issues, the political issues that need to be at the forefront and pushed forward when we're sitting at the UNSC; when we're sitting at the UN Human Rights Council in Geneva. But more so, we need to ensure that each and every one of us has this information at the tips of our hand and are able to share and disseminate facts, figures, and understanding of what is happening.

It is only because I have sat in those rooms at the UN and sat in the HRC for so many years that I have understood and seen the violent conflict of IOK. I have seen for myself.

I have been to Azad Jammu and Kashmir. I have seen how the Kashmiri people live in a safe environment, where they are protected. I felt safe and was not threatened once. I did not feel like my life was in danger or in harm. I understood because I sat and lived with the people on the ground. I sat with generations of families who have been in no contact with their families in IOK. They cried and they broke down when they could not explain in words. They could not make contact with their families that were in IOK. The number of lives that have been lost is far too many. But it is up to us now to be the voice and the reason to share what we know, because we have been there, or because we have heard the stories firsthand.

To each and every one of you, who has continued to be a part of this platform, who continues to bring voice to the IOK conflict, I applaud you and I ask you to continue doing this hard work.

To those who are on the ground and continue to suffer every single day, we keep you in our thoughts and prayers. And Insha Allah, one day, this will come to an end. In our lifetime, we will see justice; we will see that this conflict is one we talked about in the past. We will speak of it as an account of history, where we will talk of the work done by the martyrs of IOK.

How can Kashmir be granted observer status at OIC?

Catherine Constantinides:

The observer status is something that is very difficult to obtain, but it needs to be obtained via forums or civil society movements that exist.

If you have your paperwork, I would insist and encourage you to set up observer status. It is a long process to go through. Try to go through the process through your organizations or NGOs, human rights bodies etc.

The observer status is very important and it is something that we need. We must explore new avenues of collaboration, collaborative efforts across regions, across universities, across NGOs. Different civil society collaborations and coordinated efforts are extremely important. And there should be several coordinated efforts where we can talk about international solidarity campaigns, around the issue of Kashmir. We must ensure that we do all that we can, to connect with each other, and make coordination possible.

Session V

International / Internal Armed Conflicts under International Humanitarian Law

Hassan Aslam Shad[16]

We should not let these definitions and legal terminologies convolute our minds and stop us from the end goal, which is the self-determination of the Kashmiris. It is a fact that we are caught up in legal categories; I see a raging debate in the international community among Pakistanis. It's not important to categorize a conflict in a certain way.

We have the *Common Article 3* of the Geneva Conventions, which presumably applies to this situation. But the point is: IOK *is* occupied; India *is* breaching the International Humanitarian Law, and the International Human Rights Law, and even its domestic law.

Sadly, none of these things is being recognized by the international community. Thus, there *has* to be some momentum given to this struggle; there *has* to be something done differently to make it appear on the global radar for the world to see what is actually happening on the ground.

While stumbling upon some articles which had been written by international academia, I did find that there was this sort of zeroing on the freedom struggle of 1990s. The attacks in IOK constituted a violation of *Common Article 3* of the Geneva Conventions and that watered down in the future when there was a debate that perhaps this article does not even apply to the conflict today, because there is no organization of the freedom fighters.

We call them freedom fighters and the international academy refers to them as 'militants'. So, there was this sort of watering down of the rhetoric that it is no longer *Common Article*

[16] Hassan Aslam shad is Harvard Law School graduate with expertise in international law and corporate law with a heavy focus on the Middle East. Op-ed writer on law fare themes, international law, geo-strategy and international relations. Now working as Legal Director at CMS McKenna, Oman. Mr. Shad also had the distinctive honor of being the first person from Pakistan to intern at the office of the president of the international criminal court The Hague.

3 of the Geneva Conventions that applies; it is a mere internal matter or it is a situation that is governed by IHRL. So I went through those articles and in the past also I've gone through the pieces that have been written by international academics on IOK and I feel that the law is being used to deprive people of their rights. The law has become the vehicle to oppress further and that is sad, because purposes of the laws are to unshackle and to help the oppressed.

When we look at international debates that are raging on about IOK, we see that certain camps, mostly originating from India, are making a conscientious effort to dilute the freedom struggle; to make it appear as an internal struggle; that has nothing to do with the international law or its violations. Perhaps, more than anything today, we need to rewrite the IOK narrative and repeatedly demand from the international forums as well as the government of Pakistan not to treat this as a territorial issue. That claim is grounded in UNSC resolutions and has been corroded by politics.

India successfully used a narrative that Pakistan sponsors terrorism. We know that India has used this narrative for its own purposes. We need to change the prism through which we view IOK, instead of looking at it as a territorial matter. We should look at it as a humanitarian issue. We should look at it from the people's perspective. It is no longer about territory.

When I talk about the UNSC resolutions, I get an automated response that the UNSC resolutions only gave the Kashmiris the right to accede to either India or Pakistan.

I accept that. But at the end of the day we must never forget that Kashmiris as a people, stand-alone, have the right to self-determination.

A part of right to self-determination was captured in the UNSC resolutions, which gave them the right to either join India or Pakistan. But we have to look at it as an inherent issue. If we get into the granularity of the issue or to the bottom of it, we see it as a case of oppression of people's right to self-determination. That should be the thrust of the debate on IOK, and everything should lead to IHL. It will continue to be relevant because it pertains to armed conflict, and Indian military is ceaselessly violating the law. India should not and cannot dilute the right that these people have of self-determination.

We need to reconsider our IOK narrative. When I say our narrative, I mean Pakistan as well as the groups within India and within IOK itself. The Kashmiris themselves should also align and should focus on self-determination, which in itself is a stand-alone right that they are given under the international law.

Another thing that I find odd in the international community is that it is divided, on view whether IOK is India's internal matter or not. We can talk about the law; we can talk about categories; but at the end of the day, law is supposed to ameliorate the sufferings of the people. Law is supposed to take them out of the black hole, which they find themselves in. We need to look at the broader picture, the global narratives that we need to use, and the narratives that have been built against Kashmiris and Pakistan. We need to undo the minds that have been poisoned to such an extent that despite the abrogation of Article 370 and 35A on August 5, 2019, it's still taking us so much time and so much effort to sell our case before the world. And this is where we should focus and discuss IHL, the potential prosecutorial regimes available under the International Criminal Court, and other remedies that we can find ourselves.

IOK: Building a Case Under Laws of Occupation

Afzal Khushal Khan[17]

As a Research Associate at LFK, our team is constantly involved in providing legal remedies to oppressed Kashmiris, filling policy briefs on the matter, keeping a record of individuals who have been killed in occupied Kashmir, or whose human rights have been victimized by the Indian army on a daily basis.

The reason we call the territory adjacent to the Line of Control *Indian-occupied Jammu Kashmir* is quite self-explanatory. It is qualified as an occupation for multiple reasons. For instance, if we refer to *Article 42 of the 1907 Hague Regulation*, it states that a territory is considered occupied when it is placed under the authority of an hostile army.

The occupation extends only to the territory where such authority has been established and can be exercised when it comes to the IOK situation. The presence of more than 900,000 Indian forces in IOK, the atrocities committed including enforced disappearances, torture, arbitrary killings, all are on record. The presence of an hostle army is an impediment to granting basic human rights to the citizens.

According to the Common Article II of the 4th Geneva Convention of 1949, any territory occupied during international hostilities, is qualified as 'occupation of a state territory' even if there is no armed resistance. The presence of an armed resistance is not crucial to the claim that our territory is under occupation, rather the casualties of civilian Kashmiris and the hostility along the Line of Control between two high-contracting parties, Pakistan and India, is what matters and is crucial to the claim.

If a situation factually amounts to occupation, the law of occupation automatically becomes applicable, and the occupying power's confession is not needed. Since it is

[17] Afzal khushal is graduate of the University of Glasgow in international law, his thesis was on Kashmir conflict with an entire international law perspective.

primarily the law of occupation, motivated by humanitarian considerations, it is solely the facts on the ground that determine its application.

The rules of IHL relevant to the occupied territories become applicable, whenever a territory comes under the effective control of hostile foreign armed forces, even if the occupation meets with no armed resistance and there is no fighting.

That is the case of India according to Pakistan, which has *de facto* control over the territory and not *de jure*.

The communications blackout since last August is just the tip of the iceberg of the effective control that the Indian government exercises over IOK. India's control signifies an existence of a situation of occupation. Whenever a party to a conflict exercises some level of authority or control within foreign territory, under the laws of occupation, the duties of occupying power are also spelled out.

In 1907 regulations, in the articles running from *Article 42 to 56;* the four *Geneva Conventions Articles 27, 34, 47 to 78*; as well as certain provisions of *Additional Protocol 1*; and Customary IHL; the responsibility goes to Kashmiri people. The occupying power can never acquire the territory, collective or individual forcible transfers of population from within the occupied territory, and transfer of civilian population of the occupying power into the occupied territory. Be it enforced or voluntary, both are prohibited.

The abrogation of *Article 370* and the introduction of the new domicile laws are in violation of these basic responsibilities that Indian forces and the Indian government owe to the Kashmiri people.

Torture has been documented as a method of collective punishment towards Kashmiris. India is suppressing and diluting the sentiments of self-determination. Confiscation and destruction of property by the occupying power is also prohibited. All of these things are the responsibilities of the Indian government but are not being followed and hence, they're in violation of these IHLs.

As I pointed out earlier, India does not possess *de jure* control over Kashmiris. India is not the sovereign power in the territory. The *UNSC Resolution 47* defines Kashmiri people as 'people eligible for the right of self-determination'. *Resolutions 99 and 122* condemn the convening of the constituent assembly, and the addition of *Article 370* and the Indian Constitution, or the Instrument of Accession is also of little value considering questionable authority that the Maharaja possessed. He was not not elected, was unpopular, and had lost effective control of the territory because of a popular rebellion.

He signed the instrument out of pressure to rest in an unequal bargaining power with the Indian government. Reference can be made to the Vienna Convention on the Law of Treaties. It makes the instrument an unequal treaty, which tarnishes its legal validity to the colonial.

I would like to take a step back and explain the right to self-determination. It is the core issue in IOK. There is a misconception that self-determination as a right just means cessation from a territory and automatically it gives the right to a group of people to choose. However, the main issue is that the right to self-determination has two legal principles as of now, one in the colonial context and the other in the post-colonial context. It is an evolving doctrine right now, which has a link with human rights as it was encapsulated by Common Article 1 of the ICCPR and ICESCR. The colonial context definition pertains not only to *Articles 1, 2 and 55 of the UN Charter* but also the *UNGA Resolutions 1514 and 1541.*

The General Assembly *Resolution 1514* condemns the colonial relationship between the governments and affords the right to self-determination to such peoples for the first time ever. One of the provisions relates to the provision of the subjection of peoples into alien domination and exploitation, which makes colonial relationship between people and their governments illegal because, it violates fundamental human rights. Colonial rule *was* and *is* unjust. It could not be legalized, not even by plebiscite, just as slavery could not have been legalized through the consent of the slaves.

Resolution 1541 describes non-self-governing territories. The true prime factors to identify them are: first, the territory has to be geographically separated and ethically or culturally distinct from the country administering it; second, once this is established, the colonial condition is then confirmed.

That the state is administering a territory in the position of status of subjugation is happening in IOK.

According to the *1947 Independence Act*, post-British rule and partition, the right to the people is given in the colonial sense, as a territorial unit, because the right to self-determination in this context is not given to peoples, but to peoples within a territorial unit, which means: a territory can exercise its right of cessation, unlike people choosing their avenues to self-determination and choosing the destiny within a government structure.

Two things emerge from this according to the classic conception. Obviously, the people of IOK are eligible for the right to self-determination. However, the modern conception of the right to self-determination will assume that India is the sovereign over IOK, with which I strongly disagree.

However, if we assume that the right to self-determination is now applicable in the post-colonial context, if we go and adhere to the principle of *oti posedenti*, which the ICJ has used numerous times to solve territorial disputes among countries; as a doctrine it means that once independence has been exercised, borders crystallize and solidify. This is to avoid fractional and multiplication of numerous states, within a post or a country emerging from a colony.

The modern conception of the right to self-determination finds its footing in *Resolution 2625*, which states that every country and all peoples deserve the rightful determination of the principle. The resolution itself was solidified within the ICCPR in *Common Article 1* in full spirit and text. It was prescribed for all peoples. It creates a link with human rights, which exist in the times of peace. We are assuming that the Indian government is sovereign over its peoples. However, a close study of Resolution 2625, we find that there is interplay between internal and external self-determination.

Internal self-determination does not change the territorial boundaries of a state because it is an exercise within the territorial system of the state. External determination though has a three-stage meaning: it could be complete independence from that state, accession to another state, or free association with the state.

According to *Resolution 2625*, if a country does not provide its meaningful exercise of internal self-determination, it loses its sovereignty over th people. So, the self-determination is a mirror image of sovereignty of that country, if it signifies the will of those people.

In the modern context of this right to self-determination, the South Sudan case study exemplifies it. If a country does not provide for the minority rights, if it does not allow for meaningful political avenues to attain that internal determination, and if it does not protect its human rights, it loses its sovereignty. *That* is the whole argument.

Again, assuming that India is sovereign of IOK, which it is not, the Indian government loses its territorial sovereignty over IOK in the light of these arguments.

This has been alluded to by the Canadian Supreme Court in the matter of Quebec as well. They explored the concept of remedial cessation. When avenues of international determination are exhausted, and are discriminatory, which is the case in IOK, in view of the Public Safety Act and how the Indian army deals with IOK, according to the ICJ and the international law, which are neutral on the stance, remedial cessation is apt.

India is dealing with the civilian population with impunity, orchestrating and perpetrating crimes against humanity, and committing war crimes.

The Kashmiris are eligible for the right of cessation, a remedial cessation. Rather, the whole crux of this is that no matter how you spin the matter, no matter what hypothesis you pick up, the inalienable right to self-determination in the colonial context or the post-colonial context is applicable to Kashmiris.

And if we consider India sovereign, August 5, 2019 in itself, I believe, is the final nail in the coffin. Self-determination has attained the ominous character and *jus cogens* character, and it is the duty of the international community to facilitate such a right on the IOK.

The people of IOK are trying to protect their basic human rights; they seek justice in accordance with international laws they have been subjected to.

I reiterate, India's presence in Kashmir is an occupation. India owes responsibilities to the Kashmiri people and the right to self-determination does not become redundant in this process.

Indian-occupied Kashmir in Global Context: The Geopolitics of Justice

Dr. Junaid S. Ahmed[18]

We have had a lot of perspectives on the legalities on the issue. It seems fairly obvious to a decent honorable legal mind that understands international laws, what India has been doing before and now is completely against international laws. It has violated international legal treaties as well as bilateral treaties with Pakistan.

What I wanted to focus on now is: how these legal mechanisms have been insufficient until now in obtaining even a modicum of justice for the Kashmiri people? I want to focus on how the legal angles need to be joined by a host of movements and geopolitics.

International solidarity movement needs to exist among civil society social movements to express their solidarity with what's going on in IOK. We have not seen, particularly in western societies or mainstream media, if there is political and culture awareness of the Kashmir issue. The realization of occupation, and the heavily militarized nature of this occupation is absolutely absent from western imagination. Whereas, we see articles after articles, mostly written by pro-Zionists, regarding the issue of Palestine. At least, there is some form of awareness about what is going on in Palestine.

It is a situation of absolute brutality and occupation and violation of international legal treaty, but no consequences for the Zionist regime, precisely because of the geopolitics involved. It is mainly because of the uncritical blind support of the United States for what Israel is able to get away with.

What is happening there can actually offer us lessons on how to build on what we are now seeing. The recognition that what Israel is doing in Palestine is so obviously clear that

[18] He is a PhD scholar and professor of politics and islamophobia studies, visiting faculty university of Leeds research fellow center for Islam and global affairs Istanbul and the Director of the center for Muslim world studies and professor of religion and global politics.

there has been an international Zionist campaign since the June 1967 war that has tried to suppress what has been going on: the brutality of the occupation.

Israel is violating international laws, committing war crimes, crimes against humanity, and all sorts of atrocities. In the case of India, we have seen, after decades, a tilt in media coverage. This editorial shift, however, is not without reason.

There are geopolitical factors behind it. But there is also an issue within India itself: the ruling BJP, Narendra Modi, and their fascist nature. What they have been doing can just not be covered up. Over the past two years, *The New York Times* and *The Washington Post*, among others, are giving regular coverage to India's Hindutva policies.

We also see exclusive coverage on Indian-occupied Kashmir. The civil society has generated an increased awareness of the issue, which is important.

Prime Minister Imran Khan's speech at the United Nations last year was instrumental in putting this issue up on world stage, where there were people who may not have even heard of what IOK was.

We must realize that there has been an intense escalation of activism by Kashmiri journalists, scholars and public intellectuals both within and outside IOK. They have not let the issue die down.

But Narendra Modi's policies have increased the difficulties. I'm not talking about the lefties but mainstream international human rights organizations such as the Amnesty International, which say they are unable to work in Kashmir. India has become the symbol of barbarism within itself, as well as, within IOK. The conditions are just impossible to work within.

International solidarity movements with the Palestinians involve various tactics. One of them is boycotts, and sanctions, which certainly should be on the agenda, even with regards to India at this point.

We need an international solidarity movement led by the civil society, and faith-based groups. We cannot tolerate the oppression any longer! The situation demands strategies to isolate India in the international arena.

India is seen as a huge market to be taken advantage of, and hence the silence of the international community.

The recruitment of India by the United States, and by extension Israel, as a frontline state in their belligerence and containment of China has been another factor. This is geopolitics.

India is basically a partner state. It is living in a fantasy world, because actually it has become a vassal state for us.

But Pakistan too has its strengths. The two largest superpowers are dependent on Pakistan right now. The United States wants a respectable withdrawal from Afghanistan. Even the Afghan government, which has accused Pakistan for every problem the war-torn country has, acknowledges Pakistan's role in the peace process.

Then, there is this dependence of China on Pakistan. It is not a neo-colonial situation but a strategic partnership in which two powers are mutually dependent on each other. We have to realize the centrality of Gwadar port for the Chinese. US naval ships are completely encircling China. Their military bases may decide to block trade from China and its access to energy. Sino-Pak relationship is at its peak right now.

India is not fulfilling the role it was hired for. The embarrassing incident of its pilot Abhinandan Varthaman getting captured in Pakistan, and border skirmishes with China, in which it is time and again humiliated, show India's incapacity to rise as a regional power.

Even the US is increasingly reconsidering if India can rival China.

The conditions in IOK are abysmal. We have to understand the geopolitical context, and ask: how long can India sustain this? It is almost a suicidal path that the Indian state is taking. It can neither coexist with Kashmiris nor with million of Muslims in other states, and lower caste Hindus.

How long will they be able to sustain this without serious internal implosions taking place or by external social movements, civil society, faith-based groups? When movements put pressures on states, a lot of other countries get on board.

We must follow what's going on there, and link our actions in this context. Pakistan and other states must also be followed.

When Imran Khan spoke at the UN, Kashmiri activists were outside the building in solidarity. They have continued the activisim the UK, US and other countries. This issue is now in the minds of the people who had no clue about it before, and that's a huge difference.

We have the opportunity to not let it be dominated by Hindu nationalists. I will concede that I did not expect this type of coverage would be given to this issue over the past two years. So, we have to make these linkages between all of these things and yes, it *does* include geopolitics; it does include convincing and putting pressure on other states to mobilize on this issue and to see and to effectively end this.

The international community's profit-making ventures in India should not keep it from seeing Indian brutalities in IOK.

SESSION VI

Protection of Civilian Population in an Armed Conflict

Iman Zainab Hazir Mazari[19]

Even before August 5, 2019, we witnessed mass human rights atrocities in Indian-occupied Kashmir, and ceasefire violations at the Line of Control.

In the first half of 2020 alone, we have reported over 1,600 Indian ceasefire violations, while India has reported over alleged 2,400 Pakistani violations.

When these ceasefire violations result in the deaths of innocent civilians, there is a breach of the law of armed conflict, also known as the International Humanitarian Law.

Although, IHL protects all civilians, it provides for special protection of women and children, the sick, and the elderly. In April this year, there was a report of a two-year-old boy, killed during an exchange of fire between Pakistan and India at the LoC. Of course, this is in breach of the protection extended to civilians under IHL.

In the larger scheme of events, however, the illegality of these actions pales in comparison to the war crimes being perpetrated in IOK.

The *July 08, 2019 OHCHR report on the situation of human rights in Kashmir* recorded over 1,000 civilians having been killed by security forces in extrajudicial executions that occurred between 2008 and 2018.

There is also impunity for these excesses as illustrated in the fact that India has not investigated these killings, nor has had any prosecutions in this regard been reported.

---

[19] Iman mazari, LLM in international law and legal studies, university of Vienna, an international law researcher and an activist. She is also a Founding partner, MH Advocates & Legal Consultants.

Similarly, the 2019 report critiqued 'cordon and search operations', which result in large scale physical intimidation, assault, invasions of privacy, arbitrary and unlawful detentions, collective punishments, and destruction of private property.

(2) The use of indiscriminate weapons against the Kashmiri people, including pellet guns and cluster munitions by Indian security forces, represents an excessive use of force against peaceful and unarmed civilians, in violation of the UN Basic Principles on the Use of Force and Firearms by Law Enforcement Officials.

Moreover, the right to medical treatment and supplies remains a pressing concern as victims who sustain pellet and other serious injuries are often unable to obtain emergency medical assistance, particularly in light of the communications shutdown.

This is in breach of *Rule 55* of the International Committee of the Red Cross (ICRC), and rules of Customary International Humanitarian Law, which provides: *"The parties to the conflict must allow and facilitate rapid and unimpeded passage of humanitarian relief for civilians in need."*

The special rapporteur on extrajudicial, summary or arbitrary executions, in her August 2018 report titled *"Saving lives is not a crime"*, reaffirmed this obligation to allow unimpeded access to humanitarian aid and services by clarifying the implications of limitations on such access for the right to life.

In paragraph 26 of her report, she wrote: *"Acts prohibiting or otherwise impeding humanitarian services violate state's obligation to respect the right to life. Any death that may be linked to such prohibition would constitute an arbitrary deprivation of life"*. Accordingly, under IHL, States have two sets of obligations with respect to humanitarian services:

i) A positive obligation to ensure and assist humanitarian services.

ii) A negative obligation not to refuse or impede provision of humanitarian aid and services to those in need.

(3) When we speak of protection of civilians in situations of armed conflict, we do so acknowledging that there is loss of life and exploitation during times of war. The objective of IHL is to limit the exposure of civilians to exploitation, deprivation, coercion, and violence. This is why, under IHL, military considerations ought to be balanced against humanitarian requirements.

The scale, duration, and intensity of the planned military intervention must be the minimum, necessary to secure the defined human protection objective. In other words, the minimum necessary force should be utilized. Use of indiscriminate weapons is quite evidently not in line with that requirement of minimum necessary force.

While the *IV Geneva Convention Relative to the Protection of Civilian Persons in Time of War* is the relevant instrument for ascertaining the scope of protection for civilians in times of armed conflict, it is also important to understand the basic principles of IHL, which should be respected:

- Persons who are not, or are no longer, taking part in hostilities must be respected, protected and treated humanely.
- Captured combatants and other persons whose freedom has been restricted shall be treated humanely. There are special protections here against acts of violence and torture.
- The methods and means of warfare are regulated to ensure no superfluous injury or unnecessary suffering is inflicted. This is the principle of proportionality, most explicitly codified in *Article 51 (5) (b) of Additional Protocol I of 1977*, which describes an indiscriminate act as: *"An attack which may be expected to cause incidental loss of civilian life, injury to civilians, damage to civilian objects or a*

combination thereof, which would be excessive in relation to the concrete and direct military advantage anticipated". Further, in *Article 57 (2) (a) of AP I*, the notion of "precaution" is provided:

"With respect to attacks, the following precautions shall be taken: (a) those who plan or decide upon an attack shall… (iii) refrain from deciding to launch any attack which may be expected to cause incidental loss of civilian life, injury to civilians, damage to civilian objects, or a combination thereof, which would be excessive in relation to the concrete and direct military advantage anticipated".

- That the armed forces should respect the principle of distinction (contained in *Article 48 of Additional Protocol I of 1977*), which distinguishes between the civilian population and civilian objects on the one hand, and military objectives, on the other. This protection is also found in *Article 51(1) of Additional Protocol I* and *Article 13(1) of Additional Protocol II of 1977.*

Since this rule is part and parcel of Customary International Law, it applies to international and non-international armed conflicts.

Another important aspect of the proportionality principle is found in *Article 85 of AP I*, which identifies violations of AP I classified as "grave breaches" rather than "ordinary violations". Grave breaches are distinguishable from other provisions of IHL. They are considered war crimes implicating criminal liability.

In *Article 85(3)(b)* and *(c)* of *AP I*, it is stipulated: *"In addition to the grave breaches defined in Article 11, the following acts shall be regarded as grave breaches of this Protocol, when committed willfully, in violation of the relevant provisions of this Protocol, and causing death or serious injury to body or health: … (b) launching an indiscriminate attack affecting the civilian population or civilian objects in the knowledge that such attack will cause excessive loss of life, injury to civilians or damage to civilian objects, as defined in Article 57, paragraph 2(1)(iii)".*

As a general rule under IHL, civilian population and individual civilians, or civilian objects, cannot be made the targets of military attacks.

The situation in IOK, characterized as either an "occupation" which is an international armed conflict or as "non-international armed conflict", requires adherence to the same basic rules that apply in situations of international armed conflicts, including:

i) that acts or threats of violence against civilians, which are aimed at spreading terror, are prohibited;

ii) civilians only lose protection as and when they take a direct part in hostilities;

iii) starvation of civilians as a method of combat is prohibited, which includes a prohibition on attacking, destroying, removing or rendering useless foodstuffs, agricultural areas, livestock, drinking water installations, irrigation works, and similar objects;

iv) a prohibition on the forced movement or displacement of civilians.

Due to unilateral and illegal actions of India on August 5, 2019, there have been several breaches of UN Security Council resolutions, including *Resolution 47 (1948)*, which clearly states that accession of Kashmir to either India or Pakistan should be done through the democratic method of a free and impartial plebiscite.

Under *Article 49 of the Fourth Geneva Convention*, India is barred from carrying out forcible transfers of civilian populations from and within the occupied territory. It is also prohibited from transferring population from India to IOK. Since the illegal actions on August 5, 2019, any Indian can move to Kashmir, buy property there, and alter the demographics of this area, which entail consequences for any future plebiscite.

The ICJ's conclusion in its *Advisory Opinion on the Consequences of the Construction of a Wall in the Occupied Palestinian Territories,* in *paragraph 122* is of relevance here. The Court stated: *"There is also a risk of further alterations to the demographic composition of the Occupied Palestinian Territory resulting from the construction of the wall in as much as it is contributing... to the departure of Palestinian populations from certain areas. That construction, along with measures taken previously, thus severely impedes the exercise by the Palestinian people of its right to self-determination, and is therefore a breach of Israel's obligation to respect that right".*

In a similar vein, we can conclude that unilateral revocation of Articles 370 and 35A of the Indian Constitution are an attempt to obstruct the Kashmiri people's lawful exercise of their right to self-determination. This is particularly true when we look back at the UNSC's categorical rejection of Indian attempts to use the IOK Constituent Assembly to satisfy the requirement of ascertaining the will of the Kashmiri people. This is found in the *UNSC Resolution 91 (1951)* and *122 (1957)* – both of which clearly state that the final disposition of the State of Jammu and Kashmir will be made in accordance with the will of the people, expressed through the democratic method of a free and impartial plebiscite, conducted under the auspices of the United Nations.

(4) Another pertinent point to remember is the classification of India as an "Occupying Force" under IHL. To understand this, we need to address the Indian claim of legal title over Kashmir, which they ground in the Instrument of Accession.

If we accept the Indian contention that the Instrument of Accession exists, we still need to understand the nature of that instrument, which was, for all intents and purposes, a treaty of cession, i.e. a treaty under which one sovereign, having control over a particular territory, transferred title over that territory to another sovereign.

The reality is that the completion of transfer of sovereign title never occurred because the promised plebiscite never took place. Therefore, under international law, the status of the territory remains disputed and the dispute can only be resolved through a plebiscite expressing the genuine wishes of the Kashmiri people.

Therefore, India can be classified as an occupying power under international law. *Article 42 of the Hague Regulations 1907*, provides a definition of an "occupation":

"Territory is considered occupied when it is actually placed under the authority of the hostile army. The occupation extends only to the territory where such authority has been established and can be exercised".

What evidence do we have to claim that India is a "hostile army" for the purposes of this section? Well, first, there are over 900,000 troops stationed on the Indian side of the LoC, making it the most militarized zone in the world. Second, India has applied its own legal framework in Kashmir. And third, the scale of human rights violations documented in IOK, including rape, extrajudicial executions, and disappearances, reaffirm India's status as an occupying force.

The ICRC's definition of an "occupying force" deems the existence of an occupation: *"when a State exercises unconsented to effective control over a territory on which it has no sovereign title"*. Since the material condition of the plebiscite remains unfulfilled, there has been no sovereign title of transfer, which indicates that India is exercising unconsented to effective control over IOK.

In any case, there are several instruments, including the *1972 Simla Agreement*, which quite unequivocally establish that unilateral alterations of the situation in IOK shall not occur. Therefore, India's unilateral actions of August 5, 2019 are in breach of not just its multilateral obligations under the rules of IHL, but also its bilateral commitments.

Many of India's actions in IOK amount to "war crimes", which are the most serious international crimes that can be committed. There is not just state criminal liability for crimes of this nature, but also individual criminal liability, meaning: anyone who has perpetrated, ordered, organized or conspired to commit these crimes is individually and criminally liable for the same.

(5) It is unfortunate and condemnable that the atrocities and illegalities being perpetrated in IOK have been neglected by the international community, in terms of action. This is despite the fact that states, under international law, are bound not to recognize any territorial changes stemming from an illegal occupation.

This principle developed from the *Stimson Doctrine* but can now also be found in *Article 41(2)* of the International Law Commission's draft articles on the Responsibility of States for Internationally Wrongful Acts, which provide that third states (i.e. States other than India, in this case) must not recognize territorial changes resulting from annexation.

In 2015, the EU's Directorate General for External Policies provided for states to adopt the following policies in cases concerning occupations and illegal annexations, which unfortunately, we have yet to see being adopted with respect to India:

i) An unequivocal statement that the annexation will not be recognized;

ii) Prohibition of measures like investment that might support the annexation, including support for economic activity in the occupied territory under the aegis of the occupying power;

iii) Sanctions against the occupying state, particularly if that occupation is in breach of international law;

iv) Sanctions amounting to asset freeze and visa ban against those individuals who are responsible for the annexation, or who benefit from it.

The EU has, in the past, imposed sanctions in response to the illegal annexation of Crime and Sevastopol by the Russian Federation. It has restrictive measures in place targeting the import of products originating in Crimea or Sevastopol into the EU; prohibitions on infrastructural or financial investments and tourism services in Crimea or Sevastopol; prohibitions on the exports of certain goods and technologies to Crimean companies or for use in Crimea in the transport, telecommunications, energy sectors or for the prospection, exploration and production of oil, gas, and mineral resources.

Just this year, on March 16, 2020, the EU's high representative for foreign affairs and security policy stated that the EU still does not recognize the illegal annexation of Crimea and Sevastopol by the Russian Federation and continues to condemn this violation of the international law.

There is, however, visibly a double standard on IOK. Part of that double standard stems from general apathy towards the plight of Muslims in various parts of the world. And part of it is a result of the non-serious or selective attitude of Muslim States themselves towards the plight of Muslims. Another reason for this double standard rests in the fact that many Muslim countries themselves engage in human rights violations, because of which these claims are seen as mere political point-scoring.

CONCLUDING SESSION

India's Abuse of International Law: A Moment of Humanitarian Stalingrad

Muhammad Shoaib[20]

Kashmiris, for their right to self-determination, are resisting against an unwarranted and morally dull Indian occupation. The right to self-determination is a right under UN charter, where peoples of the world cannot be restricted to exercise their political fate. India is in clear contravention of international law on a number of counts; and if this drift continued the same scheme, the grail of having a potent international law system, to restrict the breach of international law, might wither away. And that is why the IOK dispute has all what it takes to be regarded as a test case for a plausible international law system, where only 'right is right' should be allowable against 'might is right'.

Indian posturing towards Kashmir dispute is against the United Nations *Resolutions 39 and 47 (1948)* respectively, and the issue of plebiscite has been totally ignored by the Indian state. But the reason why the IOK issue captivates the gravity of International Humanitarian Law is because of the significance of armed conflict in this dispute.

The Geneva Convention of 1949 proscribes employing any coercion or torture against civilians and their property, but Indian designs seem to be grounded on side stepping the invitation of IHL by exhibiting to the world that IOK is her domestic affair.

That is why, opposing the Indian draconian demeanor against IOK should not just be built upon naming and shaming their security forces who are involve in rape, torture and killing of non-combatants, but it should also be based on legally and politically countering her

[20] Muhammad Shoaib is LLM from Bahria University Islamabad under the scholarship of ICRC and his research mainly revolves around role of civilians during armed conflict. Mr. shoaib has wrote articles related to Kashmir, cpec, secp, genocide and war crimes.

illegal claim over IOK. The breaches of humanitarian laws by India, as a state flows from her occupation of Kashmiri land. Therefore, in order to meet the humanitarian concerns of the innocent people of Kashmir, the occupancy by Indian security forces shall vanish. Since the basic genesis of humanitarian abuse in Kashmir is fundamentally triggered by the Indian occupation, zero Indian occupation is the only solution to immutably safeguard the life, property and general wellbeing of Kashmiris.

International community must remember that contraventions of international law by the Indian state can be momentous and can become a majorly dangerous precedent. The ferocity and high numbers of Indian transgressions in IOK, where India alone dictates the norms of selective justice, a trend where the notion of legality is superseded by the law of the jungle and the spirit of free human conscious is suppressed by the guns and the bullets, which would eventually lead human kind to the age of force, instead of logic; reason, justice, and peaceful resolution of conflicts is not possible.

However, if the international community and international conscious acts now, and acts swiftly against India, and holds her accountable; it would send a right signal to the weaker nations and to the world in general. We would really like to keep believing in efficacy of international law, especially the IHL. And if a just resolution is reached in favor of Kashmiris, it would be a clandestine moment, similar to the battle of Stalingrad, where the Nazi defeat proved to be decisive in winning a war against a racist regime.

India's attempt to unlawfully grab land in its north and labelling it as an issue of her sovereign concern should be viewed as alarm bells and an evidence of her illegal territorial ambitions, threatening her neighbor's territorial sovereignty, and jeopardizing the peace and security in South Asia.

The role of the UNSC has to become operational now in the IOK dispute, since any delay would invite an unwarranted setting, which would eventually make the peace and security of South Asia and beyond questionable.

Oves Anwar[21]

We have a serious situation going on in Indian-occupied Kashmir. And in a battle, the other side (India) is never going to give you an inch.

There have been three wars over Kashmir while skirmishes along the Line of Control still continue. The real battle, however, the one that can produce results, is the battle of narratives, the legal battle.

Problem with the battle of narratives is that Pakistan entered the field just last year after India's unilateral actions in Kashmir on August 5, 2019. Because up until, say the 1950s and 1960s, when Pakistan was making its mark, we got UN resolutions on Kashmir, and we got some outcomes. But after that, we gave up and we forgot the rules and language of the game.

The language of the game is not shouting at the top of your lungs that Kashmir has been suffering, but through international law. Unfortunately, we have allowed our skills and capabilities to atrophy.

Therefore, we cannot even confront India when it comes to these issues. What have we been doing for the last 50 years or so, if not hiding behind our narratives and allowing the Kashmir cause to suffer?

There is a certain mentality to the actions of Pakistan, and we have to understand the psychology behind it. We are an exceptionally conservative state when it comes to the international laws. We are not willing to ratify this or that convention, treaty, or document, just out of superstitious fears. This is because we do not know how complex it is, and how

[21] Mr. Anwar is Director of Research society of International Law (RSIL). He holds an LL.M with distinction from the School of Oriental and African Studies, UK, and an LL.M in International Legal Studies from the University of Vienna, Austria. He has also earned a Diplôme d'université in International Nuclear Law from the International School of Nuclear Law, University of Montpellier, France.

to deal with it. And because of the fear, we do not even play the game and leave the field open.

And what has India done? It has taken full advantage because it has full understanding of international law, and dozens of lawyers are serving in the Ministry of External Affairs. We only have two currently, and Ministry of Law has one. The entire Pakistani state is being dealt by four lawyers with their expertise, while India has 34-50 lawyers in the Ministry of External Affairs alone. When it comes to nuclear issues, India has been able to do really well in terms of international law. When it comes to trade, India has an entire division that is able to gain advantages there, and so on and so forth. They take full advantage of their position.

One of the narratives that they have propagated is to expand the label of state-sponsored terrorism to Pakistan, and have also termed the Kashmiri freedom struggle as terrorism.

In history, every freedom struggle was initially labelled as such be it Nelson Mandela's African National Congress or the Palestine Liberation Organization. But they all had a common element that we don't: these entities voluntarily declared adherence to IHL.

The IHL is applied to high-contracting parties. High contracting parties are states. But, if you are fighting a war of liberation, you start acting like a state, start adopting the modus operandi of a state; you can start adhering to IHL obligations. Once you start adhering to them, people will start taking you seriously. The failure we have had is: we have lost capability to speak the language of international law, which is the language of international relations.

When you want a result you go to a court or a tribunal. You employ legal mechanism. We have only now begun the legal assessment of how Kashmir is under an occupation and we haven't fully built a case. The state has to take this position.

EU has certain policies when it comes to illegal annexation. What is exceptionally depressing and amusing at the same time is that Pakistan's Foreign Office is completely against the use of annexation in the conflict of Kashmir. They don't use the word annexation in the context of IOK, and I do not understand why. Using the word annexation opens up your options. If you are going to make such errors, then how can one expect India to go easy? You have your own inadequacies and lack of capacity against India.

As far as the issue of 'sovereign title' is concerned, we already know that the title is with Kashmir and not India or Pakistan. Any determination of IOK has to be done by Kashmiris. However, effective control is with India and to an extent with Pakistan. But the differentiating factor that makes India an occupying power, and not Pakistan, is the issue of hostile army, which is in the definition of what is an occupation. If Kashmiris have a sovereign title over their territory, they should be free to determine who they want on their territory. Now if that right of political determination, or the right to invite a foreign army, is taken away from them by an army, then that army becomes a hostile army.

This becomes a circular argument, which India is happy to exploit. A lot of people fell for it. The ICRC does important work, which is often not seen because it's confidential. But one problem I had working with them, and this is something that I personally felt, is that they do not want to displease India. They have their office in India, and fear New Delhi could get it folded.

When we talk about India's soft power, and we talk about its economic might, it is not just present in foreign countries; it is also very active in the international organizations. We're fortunate that after a long time, the UN was able to release two reports. Pakistan has to play on the front foot.

When we talk about crimes against humanity, we need certain basis for that. We need to start exposing individuals; through individual liability start naming and shaming individuals, including army officials. Build a case on what commands they follow, and whose commands they follow, and commit atrocities. They are investigated. The IOK police have investigated these cases but the central government under AFSPA has not given the authority to prosecute them.

Publisher: Eliva Press Global Ltd

Email: info@elivapress.com

All rights reserved.

Eliva Press is an independent international publishing house established for the publication and dissemination of academic works all over the world. Company provides high quality and professional service for all of our authors.

Our Services:

Free of charge, open-minded, eco-friendly, innovational.

-Free standard publishing services (manuscript review, step-by-step book preparation, publication, distribution, and marketing).

-No financial risk. The author is not obliged to pay any hidden fees for publication.

-Editors. Dedicated editors will assist step by step through the projects.

-Money paid to the author for every book sold. Up to 50% royalties guaranteed.

-ISBN (International Standard Book Number). We assign a unique ISBN to every Eliva Press book.

-Digital archive storage. Books will be available online for a long time. We don't need to have a stock of our titles. No unsold copies. Eliva Press uses environment friendly print on demand technology that limits the needs of publishing business. We care about environment and share these principles with our customers.

-Cover design. Cover art is designed by a professional designer.

-Worldwide distribution. We continue expanding our distribution channels to make sure that all readers have access to our books.

-Marketing tools. We provide marketing tools such as banners, paid advertising, social media promotion and more.

www.elivapress.com

Made in United States
Orlando, FL
04 November 2026

90200624R00066